The MR

(Pocket Book For Medical Representatives)

Sunil Chhabra

Books For All
(an imprint of Low Price Publications)
Delhi-110052

Distributed By:
D K Publishers Distributors P Ltd.
4834/24, Ansari Road, Darya Ganj,
New Delhi-110002
Phones: 3278368, 3261465
Fax : 3264368
visit us at: www.dkpd.com
e-mail: dkpd@del3.vsnl.net.in

First Published 2000

ISBN 81-7386-237-0

Published By:
Books For All
(an imprint of Low Price Publications)
A-6, Nimri Commercial Centre,
Near Ashok Vihar Phase-IV,
Delhi-110052
Phone: 7401672, 7452453
visit us at: www.lppindia.com
e-mail: lpp@nde.vsnl.net.in

Printed At:
D K Fine Art Press P Ltd.
Delhi-110052

The information contained in these pages has been culled from various sources. On no account should this be utilised in a lay manner. Help of a Physician/Doctor is necessary.

PRINTED IN INDIA

I owe gratitude and thankfulness to S. Avatar Singh Dua, H.P.S.E.-I (Retd.), President Ganganagar Public School, Sriganganagar, Dr. M.D. Khunger, Chandigarh, M/s. Themis Pharmaceuticals, Mumbai, Mr. Parveen Modi, B.Pharma, Hanumangarh Town, Sh. S.P. Goyal Advocate, Sriganganagar, M/s. Aarkay Computers 57, Patel Market, Sriganganagar, my wife Mrs. Suman Chhabra and one & all who were involved directly or indirectly in this venture of mine. Without them this work would not have taken its present shape.

Last but not the least, I wish to place on record my sincere thanks to M/s.Books For All, Delhi for publishing this book.

Sunil Chhabra

Foreword

To provide health care of basic as well as advanced standard is possible only by means of combined & dedicated interaction between professional of Medical Science and Pharmaceutical industry, because without this interaction the goal of providing good health to every individual can't be achieved. But in a country like India though there are various institutions & universities meant for Medical education to health professionals, but unfortunately unlike in advanced countries it is not mandatory to appear in periodic CME'S to renew the knowledge. As it is said that the Medical education has half life of only 5 years, hence it is very critical to keep the knowledge update. But in remote towns & villages of India,where Doctor have no access to Libraries or Internet, the only source is the information provided by the medical representatives.

But as to my knowledge, there is hardly any institution or syallbus & text books to prepare medical representatives for their challenging job. The only method is that every medical representative is given a short training of few days related to only those molecules which are marketed by that particular pharmaceutical house and hence there is very narrow vision of the medical representative. Though there are volumes of excellent text books in pharmacology but there was **a great need of a comprehensive book meant exclusively for medical representatives** to teach them not only the marketing aspect but also a brief introduction to medical terminology and pharmacology.

It was really exciting experience when Mr. Sunil Chhabra approached me to write "foreword" to his book entitled "**The MR**" and when I went through the whole text of book it was really a unique attempt by Mr. Chhabra who has spent lot many nights to prepare much a comprehensive, yet informative and much needed book where he had combined the marketing aspects of the job as well as the knowledge of drug and his own experience of working as a Pharma marketing professional for more than 22 years. I feel short of vocabulary to admire him and at the same time wishing him good luck.

श्रद्धावांल्लभते ज्ञानं तत्पर : संयतेन्द्रिय:।
ज्ञानं लब्ध्वा परां शान्तिमचिरेणाधिगच्छति ।।

"With devotion, one attains knowledge and through that, the control of the self. The attainment of knowledge in due course leads to ultimate peace "

Dr. L.D. Bharadwaj
M.D. (Medalist)
Sr. Consultant Internal Medicine
Bahl Hospital, Sri Ganganagar
Member National Council on
Hypertension Indian Society
Of Electrocardiology and
Cardiological Society of India

Preface

The job of a medical representative is most challenging and rewarding in nature. It gives lot of opportunities to meet different kinds of people in his daily life. Unlike other salesman a medical representative is going to promote his products to qualified experts. Apparently, he will be promoting products, but in reality he will have to sell the therapeutic ideas by persuading doctors to think towards his point of view.

To do this work successfully, the knowledge of some basic things such as nature of job, the human anatomy and physiology, the pharmacology and medical terminology is very essential. In the present volume an earnest attempt has been made to give only most pertinent information on these topics in the readable & palatable manner.

In the recent days looking to the man's renewed interest in plants as a source of useful medicines, a chapter on phytopharmaceuticals has been included in the B-section of this book.

In the recent past number of pharmaceutical companies have been introduced in the market and so many new head quarters have been created at different parts of our country for the medical representatives. Also it has been observed that most of the companies are not providing proper training to their field force. As a result number of medical representatives are facing difficulties in performing their job successfully.

This book is an effort to meet the specific needs of not only of those who are preparing to become medical representative but also of those who are actively involved in the profession.

I will feel amply rewarded if the book proves to be useful ally to a prospective medical representative, for whom it is meant. Suggestions for the improvement of this book would be most gratefully welcomed and acknowledged.

"May the auspicious dawn brighten our path and grant us wealth, vitality, wisdom and valiant posterity" - *Rigveda* *7-41-7*

Sunil Chhabra.

Contents

Section B

Chapter

Section- A

CHAPTER- 1

Medical Representative

A medical representative is a key person in marketing of pharmaceutical products. He can by his poise and grace, knowledge and sociability raise the image of his company or he can tarnish it by his illmannered or irresponsible behaviour.

In true sense he is the company's ambassador or image builder in the particular area, assigned to him by his company.

Nature of Job

The job of selling ethical pharmaceutical products is highly professional since the nature of products a medical representative deals with are technically complex.

The job of a medical representative is creative and professional in nature, and he deals with the cream of intelligensia. In fact when a medical representative succeds in developing lik'ing for his prospects and respect for him, he definitely gets more business.

On the other hand a medical representative must be well equipped with his technical information of the products which involves intensive study of pharmacology, anatomy & physiology and medicine.

In other words he must be a good salesman, who should by his salesmanship be in a position to impart his knowledge in such a way that doctors should learn without getting a feeling that they are being taught.

The medical representative is not just a commercial man, who works to earn his daily bread, rather plays a leading role by extending a helping hand to the medical profession in their taste of eradicating disease and alleviate the ailing humanity from suffering.

The medical representative's job is a dynamic one, bringing him in contact with other minds. This helps the process of mental expansion.

Every call provides a new situation, a situation which offers a real challange. It is a job to be proud of, for when the medical representative makes a success of himself, so many persons are benefited.

Qualities of a Medical Representative

(a) Physical- Sound health, Dignified posture, Proper bearing, Good nerve control, Clear voice, Neat dress, Cleanliness, Vitality and Cheerfulness.

(b) Mental- Confidence, Enthusiasm, Sincerity, Honesty, Courtesy, Tacts, Self control, Resourcefulness, Vocabulary, Sense of Humour, General Knowledge and knowledge of Current topics.

The A TO Z of Building A M.R.

A - Appearance	- Clean and proper clothing
B - Beaming	- Lightened face
C - Confident	- Always (but comes through knowledge)
D - Demonstrate	- Talk and Demonstrate with company's visual aid, product literatures
E - Enthusiasm	- Be Enthusiatic and make customer enthusiastic in buying
F - Flexible	- For better situation handling
G - Gratitude	- Reveals sincerity and honesty
H - Hard-work	- It has no substitution
I - Initiative	- Early bird catches the worm
J - Job-Evaluation	- Analyse yourself and your company's philosophy and make yourself fit for the job
K - Knowledge	- It brings confidence and enthusiasm
L - Listen	- Carefuly for better handling of objections & quaries
M - Manners	- Be courteous
N - Need	- Convert needs in to wants
O - Observant	- Watch customer buying signals & encash them

P -Planner	- First plan your work & then work your plan
Q -Question	- Ask question to get vital information
R -Remember	- The promises made and your job
S -Salutation	- Be courteous, smile naturally & shake cus tomer hand if he wants to shake your hand
T -Target	- Always determine to your objective
U -Understanding	- Make better with customer and within organisation
V -Voice	- Clear, understandable, right modulation, neither too soft nor too loud
W-Will to win	- Better sales picture
X -Exigent Attitude	- Appreciates the value of time to get better results
Y -Yearning	- Get totally involved for higher yield
Z -Zest	- For enthusiasm, to do better than others

You too can become a dynamic M.R., Check your appearance and buildup a personality which radiates enthusiasm and confidence.

Job of The Medical Representative

To create maximum demand of his company's products by visiting doctors and chemists regularly in a particular territiory or area assigned to him by his company.

"M.R. is not a salesman, but he is a marketing man, his marketing is based on the customer psychology."

Section- A

CHAPTER- 2

Salesmanship

Sale

It is the transfer of ownership in exchange of something of value, that could be a rupee/ or any other things.

Distribution

It is the physical transfer of the goods from one place to another in right quantity, of right quality, at right time, at right price and in right packing.

Salesmanship

The selsmanship is the ability of a person to handle people sucessfully.

Practically we all are salesman in this world, may be selling certain products, services or simply ideas.

It is the representative initiated effort, that provides information to the prospective customers and motivates them to make favourable decisions concerning the representative's products.

Salesmanship is a combination of both art and science. It is an art, infact a very sutler art, because it is to deal with human qualities and it is a science because it is concerned with the understanding of the principles of human nature.

John C. Brennan defiens salesmanship as "The science of understanding human desires and pointing the way to their fulfilment".

For example, even a small child knows the most effective technique to persuade his parents to buy for him a chocolate or a toy.

Thus in one way or the other every one is utilizing the principle of salesmanship.

Selling

Selling is the winning of a customer to your side, through logic and motivation. Selling is not arguing or debating.

As defined by American marketing association the selling is, "The personal or impersonal process of assisting and / or persuading a prospective customer to buy a commodity or a service or to act favourably upon an idea that has commercial significance to the seller".

Now - a - days the high pressure selling tactics to force a sale is being discouraged rather the professional marketing organisations are laying more emphasis on such type of selling that brings long term gain not only to them, but also to the customers and their field force.

Personal Selling

In the pharmaceutical industry mainly products are being promoted through their medical representatives, who visit the customers (Doctors and Chemists) regularly in an area assigned to them by their company. Thus personal selling involves a one-to-one relationship with a customer.

The personal selling is a highly distinctive form of promotion and employed for the purpose of creating product awareness, stimulating interest, developing brand preference etc.

Personal selling is the oral presentation of a tangible and intangible products by a representative to a customer for the purpose of completing an exchange.

The Selling Process

The generalised process of selling is shown & discussed below:

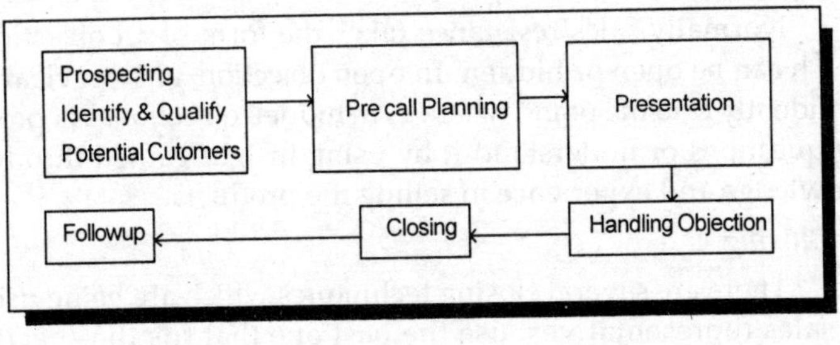

Fig.1

(i) Prospecting

The selling process begins with prospecting or finding qualified potential customer. The identification of potential customers is not an easy job, especially for a new sales representative. Rejection rate is quite high and immediate payoffs are useually minimal.

To find out most potential customers, the best sources are present customers, fellow representative, front line manager, directories, competitors & own observations.

(ii) Pre Call Planning

After identifying the most potential customer, the sales representative is to prepare for the promotion of the sale of the products. The preparation involves

(a) Gathering information in respect of customer needs and situations.

(b) Number of customers to call on that day, product slection for each customer, promotional srtategies for individual customer, etc., and

(c) To obtain permission for demonstration of the products.

(iii) Presentation

The job of a sales representative is to inform the customer about the characteristics, capabilities and availability of goods and services that are for sale.

The presentation should be interesting and clear in communication.

(iv) Handling Objections

All sales persons confront sales resistant i.e. action or statements by the customers that postpone, hinder or prevent the completion of the sale.

Normally sales resistance takes the form of an objection, which can be open or hidden. In open objection, answer clearly, confidently & to the point, where as in hidden objection, ask probing questions or understand it by using insight gained through knowledge and experience in selling the products.

(v) Closing

There are several closing techniques which are being used by sales representatives, use the best one that fits the specific prospect and selling situation.

Experienced sales representative always tries to close early. Closing is the most important aspect of the sales process.

(vi) Follow-up

The selling process is not completed by merely making the sale, follow-up after sale is an important part of whole selling process.

Effective sales follow-up reduces the customer's doubt about the product or service and improves the chance of additional sales in future.

Successful sales representative never stops serving customers. A successful salesman makes his customer, what he sell his want.

All of us being consumers often come across variety of selling situations. Differences in marketing factors cause each company to have individualised promotional strategies.

The representative has to perform a variety of different tasks and activities under different circumstances. The effective and regular sales require greater amount of creativity and perseverance, on the part of a sales representative.

"Customers do not come in search of sellers, sellers should have an eye for customers."

AIDA:- To become a successful salesman, follow the AIDA formula

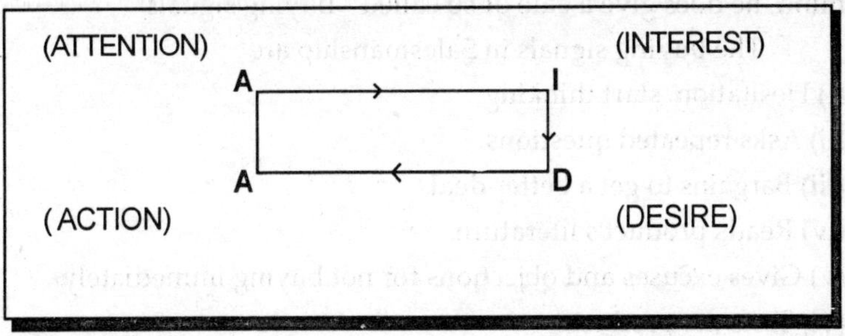

Fig. 2

A - Attention

In most of sales, the first 30 seconds play a very vital role. The representative must make a favourable impression & say the right thing at the right time.

While making the call, always be positive, cheerful and confident.

I - Interest

If there is no interest, means there will be no sale. So, find out your customer's interest and see how will your product cater for his interests.

D - Desire

Your attention plus customer's interest results in desire to purchase i.e. sales. Remember, when a customer buys, he buys for his own satisfaction. So more than selling your product, make the customer feel/ realise that this is what he wants to buy (desire).

A - Action

The way to win the battle of sale is to get an order, or commitment of your favour. Ask for the order or request for the prescription for your products. When you ask for an order, avoid asking open ended question.

Buying Signals

Try to convert needs in to wants. Be alert and watch for buying signals, which are constantly flashed at you. Whenever a customer is just convinced, but has not completely made up his mind, he does give a clue or so called " Buying signals".

The buying signals in Salesmanship are

(i) Hesitation, start thinking.

(ii) Asks repeated questions.

(iii) Bargains to get a better deal.

(iv) Reads product's literature.

(v) Gives excuses and objections for not buying immediately.

(vi) Tests the product.

(vii) Reaches for pen, and so on.

"Salesman and order booking are like bow and arrow, the nut and blot, the lock & key and like man & woman, each usless without the other."

Section- A

CHAPTER- 3

Market

Market

It is the place or geographical area for the purchase and sales of commodities in a public meeting. The market prices is the current price of a commodity.

In our country there are generally three types of market conditions

(1) Brisk (Abnormal demand for the products)

(2) Medial (Normal demand for the products)

(3) Dull (Less demand for the products)

Market Potential

It is an estimate, not a projection of the actual sales. Market potential is the maximum quantity the entire industry can sell if its marketing effort is the utmost.

But different companies might define and estimate the" number of customer", in a specific product/ market differently, even when the product is identical.

Irrespective of the product type and customers, the market potential estimation is easier when markets are well defined.

Market Demand

Market demand for a product is the total volume that would be bought by a defined customer group, in a defined territory, in a defined time period, and in a defined marketing strategies.

Market Share

Market share is the ratio of company to industry sales. It can be measured unit wise or/ and rupee wise. For example

A to z ltd. has achieved a sale of rupee 800 crores in 1998-99 and has been placed number one positon in Indian Pharma Industry.

Out of the total anti-ulcerant market, ABC brand holds maximum of 30% share.

Pharmaceutical Market

In the pharmaceutical marketing, the market is characterised by

(1) Area

It is a geographical unit demarked by boundary consisting of peoples and products of the organisation for generating business.

The medical representative is the manager of his area, who is assisted by the company's medical division, administrative department and sales department.

(2) Customers

Doctors and Chemists (Both retailers and wholesalers) and Patients (Who are indirect customers).

(a) Doctors- The town/area most potential doctors are from civil hospitals, nursing homes, private practioners and other institutions, where patients are treated or where drugs are purchased in bulk.

Doctors are the real customer for ethical products as they use them for treatment and prevention of diseases.

(b) Chemists- Include both retailers and wholesalers. These are indirect customers for pharma products, since they sell the medicines to patients on doctors prescriptions.

(c) Patients- These are also indirect customers as they purchase medicines as recommended by doctors.

(3) Competitors

That is different pharmaceutical companies.These are the interested groups who want to offer the products to satisfy the needs of the patients. Dig. representation of the pharmaceutical market:-

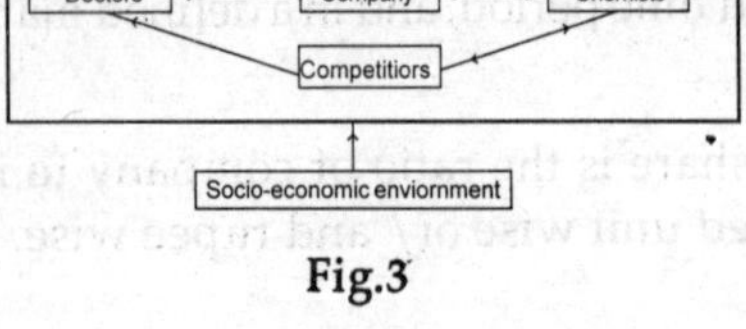

Fig.3

Thus the pharmaceutical market is made up by:

(a) Doctors- Number of doctors, their potential, location and type of practice, prescription habits, change in the prscription trends.

(b) Chemists- Number of chemists, purchasing, stocking & selling pattern of retailers & wholesalers, location, type of business (i.e. ethical/pushing/subsitution,etc.) and their financial position.

(c) Patients- Predominant diseases & incidence of prevalence thereof', purchasing capacity, population of the town (area).

(d) Company- Image & reputation of your company, movement of company's products overall.

(e) Competitors- Competitive activities including number of medical representatives, image & reputation of competitors, promotional strategies of the competitors.

(f) Socio-Economic Environment- Factors having impact on demand & sales.

So the pharmaceutical market is the place where exchange of resources takes place between the company and patients, through their purchase of medicines from retailers(and wholesalers), being influenced by the doctors.

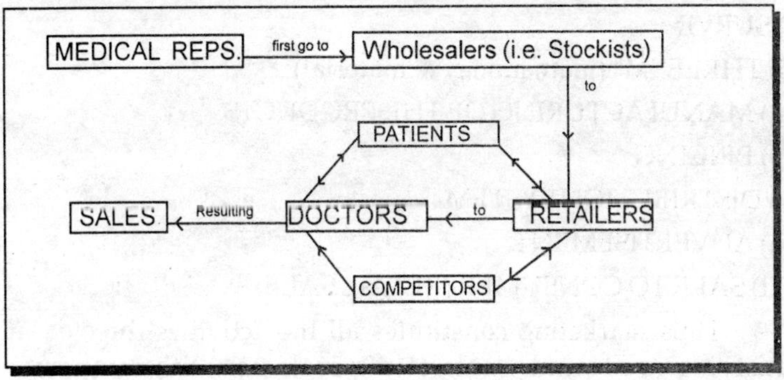

Fig. 4

"First arouse in the other person an eager want, he, who can do this has the whole world with him, he, who cannot walks a lonely way."

Section- A

CHAPTER- 4

Territory Marketing Management

Marketing

When ever a businessman want to start some manufacturing business i.e. to manufacture some products the function of the marketing starts. In other words right from concieving the idea of manufacturing a particular product, till the time it is being consumed or used by the consumer, all the steps which the product has to pass through are called "MARKETING".

To be more precise, following are the function of the marketing:

(i) SURVE

(ii) THREE "M" (man, money & material)

(iii) MANUFACTURING OF THE PRODUCTS

(iv) PRICING

(v) DISTRIBUTION SYSTEM

(vi) ADVERTISEMENT

(vii) SALE TO CONSUMER (RETAIL SALE)

Thus marketing constitutes all the activities directed at satisfying needs and wants of the customer with company's product.

Management

It is the functional process for planned and efficient utilisation of resources to get the desired/ optimum results.

Marketing management is extension of the management processes in marketing activities.

Medical representative is the most important link in the company's operations through which, the company activates, directs and fulfills the exchange (marketing) process.

Dig. presentation of marketing management:-

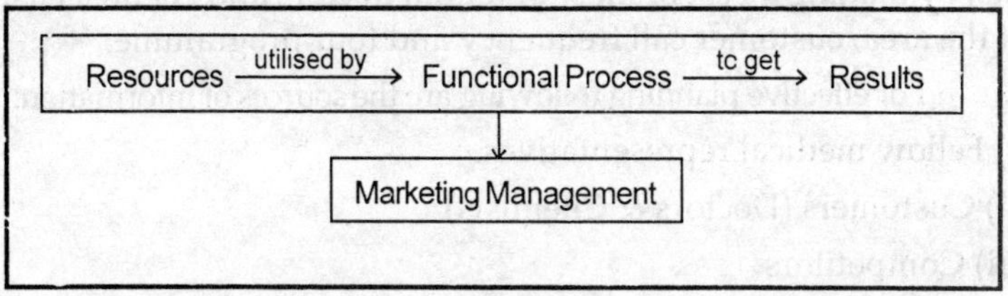

Fig. 5

(a) Resources

In pharmaceutical selling marketing resources are medical representatives knowledge, skills, time and promotional tools.

(b) Functional Process

Functional process means the planned and efficient utilisation of resources.

Dig. representation of functional process:-

Planning — Implementation of plans — Assessment — Field Information system

Fig. 6

(i) Planning

Planning ensures achievment of desired goal , through undergoing all actions required in a given situation.

In pharmaceutical market doctors needs, patients needs and chemists needs keep on changing. Also socio-economic factors and competitor's activities affect sale. So one should understand the present status and changing trends at the market place.

Planning plays a positive role in the selling process and is a vital selling tool. It gives conviction, generates confidence and enthusiasm.

Development of a plan for an area, includes the following sub-plans:

(a) Customer coverage plan

It is a plan of optimising results through effective coverage of customers. (i.e. Doctors & Chemists.)

This includes customer selection i.e. Doctors and Chemists, by making a best of most potential doctors and chemists list of the area, customer call frequency and tour programme.

For effective planning following are the sources of information:

(i) Fellow medical representatives.

(ii) Customers (Doctors & Chemists)

(iii) Competitors

(iv) Trade associations

(v) Own company feed back.

(vi) Trade directories

(vii) Railway and Bus Time Tables.

(viii) Observations

The purpose of the customer coverage plan helps

(i) To communicate product promotional message to maximum number of doctors. Only doctors can contributes towords increased demand of the company's products month after month.

(ii) To decide on the number of doctors who can be called on effectively on that day/ month, by utilising the available resources to get maximum returns from doctors covered.

(iii) To set a call frequency which will yield the optimum results.

(iv) To determine the number of retailers and wholesalers to be covered on that day/ month, to ensure availability of company's products in adequate quantities at all times, so that prescriptions generated are fully encashed.

(v) To collect vital information on prescription habits of doctors, movement of company's product as well as that of competitors, competitors activity, etc.

(vi) To achieve customer coverage in the most economical manner possible.

For examples:

(i) XYZ company's head office circulate a circular directing their Medical Representatives to call on 135 doctors once a month and 60 most potential doctors at his head quater twice a month.

It means app. 12 day's are required for working at head quater and another 12-13 day's for working at ex. head quater & out-station towns. He must plan his monthly tour-programme in such a way that he is able to cover all the customers in a month as per the directives of the company, in a most economical manner possible.

(ii) One of the suggestive plan can be- A medical representative has made a plan to callon suppose 12 doctors and 6 retail chemists at his town of head quater on a particular day.

It will be ideal for him to further plan all the 18 calls situated in the same area or near by areas, to ensure effective coverage within limited time framework.

(b) Plan for implementation of promotion

In pharmaceutical selling,face to face detailing of products is the most effective method of communicating company's products information to the doctors. Only doctors can contribute towards increased demand of the company's products.

Effective communication of the promotional message in accordance with the indiviual doctor's needs & situation is the essence of a good detailing. For the effective implementation of product promotion, the medical representative should have the background information in terms of

(i) Complete product knowledge

(ii) Communication skills

(iii) Individual doctor's prescription habits and company's products plan thereof'.

(iv) His promotional tools plans for individual doctor's

(v) Appropriate time plan for each call.

(c) Plan for the achievement of area sales target

Budget and Target - Budget is a working plan for one year, whereas target is a goal.

To achive the area sales target, first break-up the annual target in to quarterly, monthly and then on daily basis. Once daily sales plan is planned for each product & Rs. wise, orders from stockists should be booked in adequate quantities for each product. Then daily personal order booking from retail counters should be planned to meet the incremental prescription demand expected from selected doctors of that area, locality.

Now, the promotional activity should generate demand not less than, what was planned for that particular day. Plan for daily achivement, will also provide opportunity to take corrective steps well in time.

(ii) Implementation of plan

The optimum/ desired results can be obtained through effective implementation of the plan. This could be possible only when medical representative realises the importance/significance of each activity planned for the achievement of set targets.

For this a medical representative must possess the following primary requirements in his own:

(a) Knowledge (b) Punctuality (c) Determination

(d) Skills (e) Organising of daily work

(f) Observing capability.

Implementation of the daily plan must utilise all avaliable resources & efforts to achieve area/ town wise daily sales plan.

(iii) Assessment

It is very much essential to assess the achievement v/s plan made for that day/ month, on a regular basis.

This assessment should include all areas, viz:

(a) Sales plan v/s Achievement

(b) Field activity (Customer coverage plan v/s Achievement)

(c) Promotional plan v/s Achievement

Based on the achievement (positive or negative) compared to plan made, a revision in the plan becomes necessary to ensure achievement of monthly/ yearly sales plan well in time.

(iv) Field Information Systems

The field information systems forms the basic backbone of planning and improving field activity. It provides a firmer grip on an area & helps in the improvement of existing products & in introducing new products.

The field information is a yard stick to measure results v/s efforts.

For gathering field information, the company (s) provides various instruments such as:

(a) Doctor list

(b) Chemist list

(c) Daily / Biweekly reports

(d) Monthly report

(e) Daily work diary, etc.

Reporting- The M.R. plays the role of eyes and ears of the organisation he represents. The report and reporting system help a medical representative and his company as it

(i) Increases efficiency through scientific recording.

(ii) Improves the coverage of customers.

(iii) Measures results v/s efforts.

(iv) Helps in the improvement of existing products and in the introduction of new products

(v) Helps to give services and improve the sales through timely follow-up.

(vi) Helps to improve selling techniques.

(vii) Saves time for the planning.

(viii) Helps the M.R. to keep abreast of territory development.

(ix) Focuses attention on additional duties and reminds the M.R. to perform them.

(x) Helps to analyse lost sales.

(xi) Keep tabs on competition.

For a report to be effective and meaningful; it should fulfil following:

(a) It must be submitted on time as otherwise it has only histori cal value.

(b) It should be accurate and must present facts as they have/are happening.

(c) It should be specific and, not unnecessarily long.

(c) Results

In pharmaceutical marketing, the results are expressed in terms of

(i) Sales achievement

(ii) Growth rate of products & market share

(iii) Customer coverage

(iv) Customer relations

(v) Expense control/profit, etc.

These are further broken in to zone-wise, region-wise, area-wise, territory-wise and are co-ordinated with the help of the various departments of the company.

The M.R. can up date himself with all these by going through the company's promotional strategies, detailing aids, product manuals, through communication with senior managers and by participating actively in sales meetings and training programmes.

" The man who can benefit most of all from his own analysis and study of his reports is the prospering salesman"

Section- A

CHAPTER- 5

Communication

Communication has a variety of roles to play. It brings the communicator and receiver closer to each other in their desire to acheive their respective goals.

For example a marketing company has such goals as Profitability, Corporate credibility and Market leadership. Similarly, consumer too have such goals as better consumption, staying informed on new buying alternatives and a desire for a better quality of life.

Communication is a dialogue and not a monologue between communicator and receiver. The communication can be conceptualized at both macro and micro levels. Broadly defining-"Communication is a well planned and tactful action directed to get desired results".

Basic law of Communication

(1) The communicator must communicate (speak up). He must have something to say, the ability to say, the courage to say, in a tactful manner.

(2) Good communication is always well prepared.

Ways of Communication

In a wakeful day we are spending times for communication like this:

(i) WRITING	7 TO 10%
(ii) READING	10 TO 15%
(iii) SPEAKING	30 TO 35%
(iv) LISTENING	40 TO 50%

Listening is an active communication process. Almost 45% of our wakeful hours, we spend listening and just about 30% of speaking. Much of what we learn is obtained through good listening.

Listening is not just hearing. The hearing is done with the ears and listening is done with mind. It is a skill and requires development on regular basis. Always try to think in terms of other person's interests, be alert and don't assume any thing. Evaluate during listening and hold out your judgement till the other person completes his talk.

Ask question in a permissive fashion. Sit alert, leaning forward, maintain eye to eye contact, don't cross your arms and legs, don't look tense, be relaxed, carefully watch person's body language and don't indulge in or encourage side talk during the call or meeting.

Process of communication

Diagrammatic representation of the process of communication

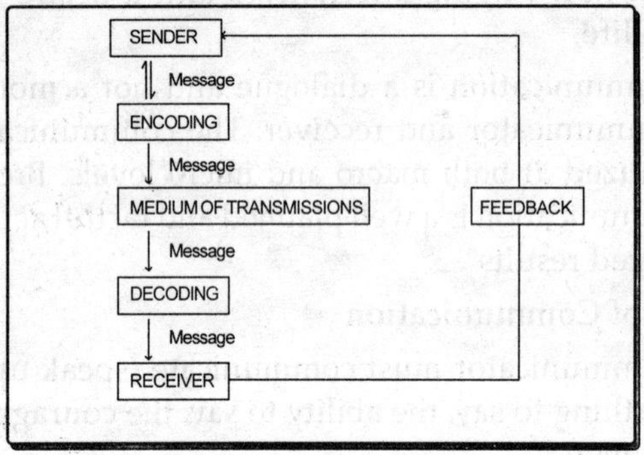

Fig.7

The basic elements of communication are:

(i) The sender (source) who is the orginator of the message.

(ii) The receiver, who is the ultimate destination of the message

(iii) The medium of transmissions, the means by which the mes sage moves from sender to receiver.

These elements are joined together by a process which includes " enconding " (put in an understandable form) and "decoding" (retranslation into understandable terms). The feed-back is an indication of understanding all the message, by the message receiver to the message sender.

Why communication fails

(i) Communicator doesn't care.

(ii) Communicator viewed as routine activity.

(iii) Problem of day to day life interfere with the communication process.

(iv) If a person makes a long gap with receiver.

(v) Natural differences in understanding between communicator and receiver .

(vi) Sound Pollution.

Rules for Good communication

(i) Well planned wording.

(ii) Positive listening attitude.

(iii) Strong & able leadership.

(iv) Answering questions & objections.

(v) Frankly admitting "No".

Marketing Communication

In pharma industry for a vary long time, it had been seen that promotions formed the only communication-bridge between a company and its customers. This limited view of marketing communication is now being replaced with a more correct and wider proposition, that marketing communication travels beyond promotion. In its linkages with customers, it encompasses every thing including - product, packaging, distribution channels, services and forms as a vital part of overall marketing efforts towards customers and also the other section of society.

Marketing communication can be define as " The continuing dialogue between customers and company in a market place".

Role of Marketing Communication

(i) Establishes company's image/or prestige.

(ii) Communicates features of products and services.

(iii) Creates awareness for new products and series.

(iv) Keeps existing goods and services popular.

(v) Generates enthusiasm.

(vi) Convinces customers.

(vii) Justifies prices of the products and services.

(viii) Provides after sale services for customers.

The marketing communication comprises of several elements viz. Advertising, Publicity, Packaging, Personal selling, Sales Promotion, etc.

In pharmaceutical marketing, communication is being made through detailing by the Medical Representative to the customers (mainly doctors) with the help of promotional tool like products' literature, visual-aids, etc., and plays an important role to develop sales picture of the company.

Detailing

In pharamaceutical selling, face to face detailing of products is the most effective method of communicating company's products information to the doctor's. Thus detailing is the "Sum total of all activities involved in generating prescription".

The Importance of Good Detailing

Good speech enhances personality. It will put you ahead above the crowd and may well pave the way for promotion and greater security.Please check, when you speak do you mutter, or grunt, or whisper, or bellow ? Are you understood first time ? Is your voice attractive ? If it is not, then try to improve your weakness.

For example - one way to improve the weakness, is that he should read detailing notes or newspaper loudly, by sitting infront of a mirror in a closed room. He should do it time and again till he cures his weakness/ shyness.

People judge you by your voice and the quality of your speech. So dress your detailing well and see that it attracts doctors rather than repels.

Types of detailing

There are several types of detailing styles, few common one are:

(i) Persuasive (Influencing the customer by arguments, may win the battle)

(ii) Assertive (Self confident, act positively & detail as directed/trained)

(iii) Bridging (Supportive talk,lack of confidence and enthusiasm)

(iv) Attractive (Confident, knowledgable talk, offer better services, open and close the talk in a impressive way)

Things Required for an Effective Detailing

(i) Products literature or visual aid and its handling.

(ii) Speed of detailing .

(iii) Pitch of voice.

(iv) Modulation of voice.

(v) Stress and pause.

(vi) Point out .

(vii) Eye to eye contact.

(viii) Body language .

(ix) Continuity.

(x) Impressive closing.

The good detailing must incorporate followings:

A - Attention to Problems

S - Solution to Problems

P - Product for the Solution of Problems

I - Information of the Products

C - Closing

Why Detailing to Doctors

As discussed earlier, in pharmaceutical marketing face to face detailing of the products is the most effective method of communicating merits of the products. Effective detailing favourably influences the doctors' thinking towards your products and resulting in maximum number of prescriptions in favour of your products.

"Doctor chooses not between products, but between personalities,"

Section- A

CHAPTER- 6

Handling Objections

It is very well said that "The sale really begins when the customer says no". The wants of an individual can be unlimited, but on the other hand, purchasing power has definite limitations. A sales presentation can lead to silence, questions, agreement, or objections.

Most of the medical representatives walk out of a sales call very happy, that the customer gave them a patient hearing and not raised any question or objection. In the absence of sales resistance the M.R. believes that sales is being made. Infact, such sale calls are poor calls and generally are non-productive. It only shows that the customer has not been stimulated to buy and hence has not asked any question to fully satisfy himself about the product (s), which a M.R. is trying to sell.

Objections

An objection is an argument legitimately offered in good faith by the customer, under conditions in which the customer is still undecided and anxious to find the correct answer for his needs.

An objection is a valid request for further information. It is difficult to conceive of a sale pursued from the beginning to the end without encountering some such request.

The starting point is to make difference between an objection and an excuse. When ever a customer makes an excuse, it is insincere resistance designed to get rid of you, for it also shows total lack of interest.

So one must identify the difference between an excuse and an objection through keen observation and judicious interpretation.

Watch carefully the words and the tone of the customer. Ask tactful questions to get the useful clues and must see the customer's need as our need.

Why do Customers raise objections ?

(i) Less understanding

(ii) Inadequate information

(iii) Inaccurate information

(iv) Habit - reluctant to change, etc.

Very often customers raise objections because they have not really listened during sales call. Thus, constant involvement of the customer is required to ensure that the right message is going across to him.

Thoughts on objections

(i) It shows that customer is expressing a desire to buy.

(ii) Each objection is one step forward.

(iii) They show that some progress is being made step by step.

(iv) There is nothing objectionable about an objection, but there may be more to answer to it.

(v) Successful handling means greater confidence.

If the presentation is well organised and planned, the customer may not raise difficult objections. Objections of quality, price, delivery, discount etc. reflect customer's interest. It is an excellent opportunity for the M.R. to start a dialogue with the customer and know what is really stopping the sale.

Therefore, it is better to have a customer who raises objections rather than one who keeps silent .

Types of objections

(a) Resistance to change

People normally resist change, which results in the form of an objection. To meet this situation the M.R. must project his sales talk in such a way that the customer sees 'advantages' in switching the product.

(b) Lack of understanding

It is a human failure. The customer either misunderstands or becomes confused about the selling proposition. A clear and precise sales presentation will help to reduce this form of sales resistance.

(c) Objection to price

The product price is always important to the customer. Hence every sales person must expect his price to be challenged and must be able to defend it.

(d) Emotional reactions

Emotion is almost always present when there is sales resistance. Occasionally it can be either the customer is provoked against the M.R. & / or his company, or the customer may have his own personal problems.

How to meet objections

The ability to meet an objection that is raised by the customer during the course of the sales call, is an invaluable asset to a M.R. and it requires

(i) Ability to listen and encourage customer to speak.

(ii) Knowledge of the customers, products, competition and salesmanship.

(iii) Representative's interest.

(iv) Cool yet sharp business like temperament.

(v) Ability to convincingly communicate, without arguing.

(vi) Inoffensiveness on the part of representative.

Suggested steps to overcome objections

Objections or sales resistance are a common part of a medical representative's life. Don't be worried about objections. Don't be rattled by them. Tackle them with confidence and more often than not, if a M.R. has the requisite product knowledge, the objection can be converted into a sale. Below written are some direct or indirect suggestive steps to overcome objections

(i) Listen carefully before answering.

(ii) Pay due respect to the customer and his problem.

(iii) Postpone answeing immediately, it may be covered up in the subsequent presentation.

(iv) Repeat the objection in statement or question form (This will satisfy the customer with an assurance of your understanding of his problem).

(v) Do not lecture or argue.

(vi) Highlight benefits and show what delay costs.

(vii) Break the question/objection into segments.

(viii) Comparison of products - stress your plus points.

(ix) Give proof or guarantee for quality and service.

(x) Use third party evidence.

(xi) Offer a trial.

(xii) Ask questions.

(xiii) Let it bounce back.

(xiv) Ignore-if it is a trifling objection, it will not be repeated.

(xv) Finally, you can answer objections only if you know the answers.

"Try honestly to see things from the other person's point of view."

Section- A

CHAPTER- 7

How To Become a Star Representative

When a medical representative visits a doctor or chemist, a mental picture is formed about the company, he represents. Their are mainly two types of medical representatives - one is ordinary and another is professional. The basic difference between them are as

ORDINARY M.R.	PROFESSIONAL M.R.
(1) Works haphazardly and without a pain	(1) Work systematically. He first plans his work and then works his plan.
(2) Price conscious	(2) Thinks of values and benefits.
(3) Rarely confident	(3) Very much confident.
(4) Only writes what he is told	(4) Creates an urge to buy.
(5) Blames everybody and anything for his failure	(5) Tries to find out his own faults by analysing his work.
(6) Takes no as final answer & walks away.	(6) Takes no as a challenge and sells better.

"Order ensures early success discipline ensures long term service"

The most important quality of a star Medical Representative is a positive thinking.The M.R. who has a positive mental attitude will learn to over come most difficult hurdles. He knows how to make things happen.

To become a dynamic sales-personality, a medical representative must have the following qualities:

(i) Should wear clean and proper clothes.

(ii) Confident, Jolly and cheerful.

(iii) Enthusiastic.

(iv) Friendly without being familiar.

(v) Honest and sincere to his company.

(vi) Keen and courteous.

(vii) Positive thinker.

(viii) Tactful.

(ix) Sharp memory .

(x) Clear voice

What is the secret of a star medical representative

Why he gets more success when other fails? A star medical representative makes all his efforts to be a professional. This he does by doing the followings

(i) Checks stock position of his products as well as of his competitors before the start of his work

(ii) Well equipped with knowledge that further brings confidence and enthusiasm.

(iii) First plans his work and then works his plan.

(iv) Hard-worker.

(v) Sincere & honest.

(vi) Determined to his objectives.

(vii) Will to win, demonstrate the benefits of his products to the customer's satisfaction.

(viii) Positive thinker

(ix) Flexible.

(x) Listens carefully, handles complaints, answers quarries and over comes objections.

(xi) Analyses situation and corrects himself accordingly.

(xii) Asks questions- for customer attention and gets the vital information.

You too can become a star sales personality. It is in your hand to make your customer like you, accept you and do business with you.

"M.R.S. are not born but they are made by scientific learning"

Section- B

CHAPTER- 1

Organisation Of The Human Body

The Human Body

The human body is composed of microscopic living units called the "cells". Cells of one type collect together and form a "tissue".

Different tissues take part in the formation of an "organ" (e.g. Heart, lung, Stomach, etc.). A number of organs form a "system", which is designed to carry out a specific function.

Number of systems for example, the circulatory system, the urinary system, the musculo -skeletal system, the nervous system, the digestive system, the reproductive system, etc. form the human body.

To describe the human body and its various parts, certain terms are frequently used as written below:

Ventral	:	The front aspect of the body.
Dorsal	:	The rear aspect of the body.
Anterior	:	The part which is towards the front.
Posterior	:	The part which is towards the rear.
Superior	:	The part which is towards the head.
Inferior	:	The part which is away from the head.
Medial	:	The part which is towards the mid-line.
Lateral	:	The part which is away from the mid-line.
Proximal	:	The part which is attached closer to an organ.
Distal	:	The part which is attached away to an organ.

Surface landmarks

Certain terms are commonly used to describe various areas on the anterior surface of the trunk. For example in describing the location and symptoms, there are nine areas of the abdomen viz. two hypochondria, two lumbar regions, two iliac fossae, an epigastrium, an umbilical region and a hypogastrium, as shown in fig. -8.

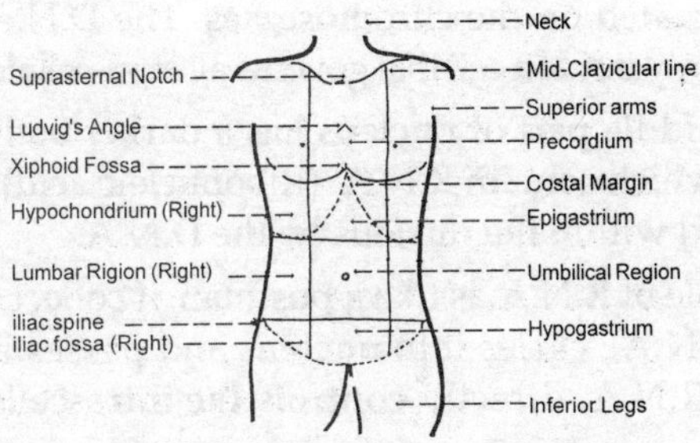

Surface Landmark and areas on the ventral surface of body.

Fig. 8

It is important to study the cells, its structure and functions. This will enable us to know about the construction of human body, its functions and how it is influenced by disease as well as how drugs cure the disease.

Whatever changes occur in the human body, can be traced at the cell level, where the ultimate events take place.

The Cell

A cell is a small microscopic structure looks like a tiny bag of living substance called "protoplasm" which is enclosed in a thin membrane called "cell membrane".

The protoplasm consists of "cytoplasm" and a dense body called "nucleus".

(i) Cell Membrane

It is a thin covering madeup of protein and the fat molecules. It controls the movement or permeation of substances into & out of the cell.

Cell membrane also contains specific receptors for drugs, i.e. points of contact for certain drugs.

(ii) Nucleus

It is a dark body found almost in the centre of the cell. Nucleus contains "Chromatin", which gives rise to "Chromosomes" during cell division. The chromosomes are 46 in number in human being [arranged in 23 pairs] and are fine thread like structures.

Chromosomes are rich in D.N.A. (Deoxyribonucleic acid) & are carriers of hereditary information." Genes" are the information units situated on the chromosomes. The D.N.A. is also the highest authority inside a cell that governs all intra-cellular functions.

The middle part of nucleus has a darker body called the" Nucleolus" which contain R.N.A. (Ribonucleic acid). The R.N.A. is synthesised within the nucleus by the D.N.A.

The role of R.N.A. is like a postman, it collect the information from D.N.A., caries it to nucleus and passes it on to cytoplasm. The R.N.A. directly controls the intra-cellular protein synthesis.

(iii) Cytoplasm

The cytoplasm contains a number of specialised structures known as "organelles", as written below:-

(a) Golgi-Body

It is situated near the nucleus, comprising of several closely packed tubules. The golgi body concentrates the cell's secretions.

(b) Centrosome

It is situated just outside the nucleus and contains two "centrioles". The centrosome plays an important role in cell division.

(c) Mitochondria

They are called power house of cell. These oblong structures have shelf-like projection inside and contain enzymes which metabolise food stuff and release energy required for the cell's activities.

(d) Endoplasmic Reticulum

This is a network of fine tubular structures. Some of them are " smooth" and contain the "microsomal enzyme", which metabolise drugs. Other form carry "granules" along them, called "ribosomes", which contain R.N.A. and are the centres for protein synthesis. The synthesised protein mostly acts as enzyme.

(e) Lysosomes

They are dark bodies, rich in enzymes. The lysosomes disrupt when the cell is injured or damaged and release enzymes that digest the non-viable cell and help its disintegration and disposal.

Besides the above the cytoplasm also contains proteins, fats, glycogen, secretion of the cell and waste products.

Cell Division

There are two types of cell division, occurs in the body:

(1) Mitosis

Normal cell division occurs in the body in which one cell is divided in to two small similar structures, called the daughter cells containing the number of chromosomes equal to that of the parent cell. Mitosis consist of four phases, viz. Prophase, Metaphase, Anaphase and Telophase

(2) Meiosis

It occurs in the primary sex organs i.e. ovaries and testies to form ova and spermatazoa respectively. Here the daughter cells contain only half of the number of chromosomes of the parent cell.

When an ovam is fertilized by a spermatozoon the original number of chromosome is restored, each contributing one-half. The sex of a child depends upon the union of "X" or "Y" sex chromosomes of the father with the "X" sex chromosomes of the mother within the ovum.

Types of Cells

The single cell organisms such as Amoebae performs all essential functions, but in highly developed and complex organisms, cells under go specialisation so that they are better equipped to carry out one function. For example -gland cells secretes, smooth muscle cells contract & relaxe, nerve cells conduct impulses, etc.

Functions of Cell

A living cell performs several essential functions in the body , these are Nutrition, Metabolism, Excretion, Respiration, Growth, Reproduction, Auto-regulation and Excitability.

The Tissues

A tissue is the group of one type of cells. There are mainly four types of tissues:

(1) Epithelial (2) Connective

(3) Muscular (4) Nervous

(1) Epithelial Tissues

The epithelial tissues form lining of body surface & body cavities. The cells of epithelial tissues are closely packed with minimum intra-cellular space or substance. They may be flat, cubical or columnar in shape and have a remarkable ability to multiply and replace damaged or dead cells.

(i) Simple Epithelium- The epithelium consisting of single layer of cells, is called "simple `epithelium" , e.g. Squamous, Cuboidal, Glandular, Columnar, Brush-Border and Ciliated, etc.

(a) Squamous Epithelium- The flat, scale-like cells arranged in a single layer. Found in the lining of heart, blood vessels and body cavities.

(b) Cubical Epithelium- It is found in the ducts of glands, for example, in the glands, pancreas, sweat gland and lacrimal glands. Also known as "Glandular epithelium".

(c) Columnar Epithelium- It is found in the lining of the stomach, the inestines and the kidney tubules. "Brush-Bordered" which are found in the intestines, "Gobletells" are found in the stomach & "Ciliated "are found in the urinary tubes and the respiratory passage.

(ii) Compound Epithelium

The epithelium consisting of many layers of cells, is called "Compound epithelium", e.g.- Transitional and Stratified, etc.

(a) Transitional Epithelium - It is found in the lining of the ureters,the urinary bladder & the urethra.

(b) Stratified Squamous Epithelium- It is found in the mouth and the gullet. The epidermis (outer layer of skin)is also a stratified squamous epithelium,consisting of five distinct layers viz.- horney, clear, granular, thorny & basal layer.

The epithelia which line body cavities are supported on a bed of connective tissues to form a membrane.

The membrane which line cavities open to the exterior are called "mucous membranes"(e.g. mouth, gut, nose, vagina), which produce mucous.

The membranes which line closed body cavities are called "serous membranes" (e.g. pericardium, pleura, peritonium) and membranes which line joint spaces are called"synovial membranes", they produces a thick glairy fluid that lubricates the joint surfaces.

(2) Connective Tissues

The connective tissue provides frame-work, support or packing material for other tissues.It is characterised as a small number of cells with a large intervening matrix,cementing substance or medium. Examples are the blood,fibrous tissue,reticular tissue,elastic tissue,adipose tissue,cartilage and bone.

(i) Blood- This is a connective tissue containing R.B.C.,W.B.C.and Platelets in a fluid medium called as plasma.

(ii) Reticular Tissue- This is found in spleen, lymph nodes and bone marrow and having semi-solid matrix.

(iii) Fibrous Tissue- They have semi-solid matrix and contains two types of fibres, the "collagen fibres" and the "elastic fibres".The fibrous tissue may be loose or dense.

The loose fibrous tissue is found between organs and forms the sheaths of nerves, muscles & blood vessels.

The dense fibrous tissue is strong and forms the ligaments. The cords of dense fibrous tissue which attache muscles to bones are called tendons.

(iv) Elastic Tissue- They differ from fibrous tissue and found in the wall of blood vessels, wind pipe and in some ligaments of the joints of the back-bone.

(v) Adipose Tissue - It serves as cushion for various organs, an insulating layer under the skin and a reserve of food.

(vi) Cartilage- It has solid but resilient matrix.It is of three types-the"hyaline cartilage"found at the ends of bones at joints, the "white-fibro cartilage "found between the vertebrae and the"elastic cartilage"found in larynx and external ear.

(vii) Bone- The hardest connective tissue having rigid and solid matrix. The bone tissue is of two types, the "spongy", found in the vertebrae, skull bones, wrist, ankle, ends of long bones and the"compact", found on the surface of all bones and forms the shaft of long bones.

(3) Muscular Tissues

The cells of muscular tissues are elongated and capable of contraction and relaxation. e.g. smooth muscles, skeletal muscles and cardiac muscles tissue.

(i) Smooth Muscles- These muscles are also known as unstriped, visceral or involuntary muscles. They consist of elongated spindle shaped cells with a central nucleus. They undergo spontaneous, slow rhythmic contractions under the influence of the autonomic nerves. These are found in the walls of blood vessels and viscera i.e. internal organs, such as stomach.

(ii) Skeletal Muscles- These muscles are also known as voluntary, striped muscle and found in limbs, neck and trunk. They are capable of quick, powerful and sustained contractions under the influence of voluntary or somatic nerves.

(iii) Cardiac Muscles- They consist of branching, striated cells connected with one another to form long fibres. These muscles are endowed with a capacity to generate impulses spontaneously, which are responsible for the heart's rhythmic contractions and relaxations.

(4) Nervous Tissues

The basic units of nervous tissues are called "neurones" (Nerve cells). Besides there are inactive, supporting cells called as "neuroglia" or glial cells, The neurones are of three types

Sensory Neurones	-	Carry impulses from various tissues & organs to the brain.
Motor Neurones	-	Carry impulses from the brain to the or gans and tissues.
Associated Neurones	-	Carry impulses between various neurones.

The nerve cell consists of a cell body with nucleus and two kinds of processes - "dendrites", receive impulses and "axons", carry impulses away.

The neurone has the power of excitation and conduction.

Organs and Systems

Various tissues take part in the formation of an organ

(Stomach, Heart, etc.) and the organs in turn are associated meaningfully to constitute the body systems (The digestive system, the urinary system, etc.) The details of organs & systems are descirbed in the subsequent chapters.

Basic Medical Sciences

Anatomy- The study of structure of the human body by means of dissection.

Histology- A subdivision of anatomy, which deals with the microscopic structure of the tissues & organs.

Physiology- The study of body functions.

Bio-Chemistry - The study of chemical reactions taking place in the body.

Microbiology- The study of microscopic living organisms.

Parasitology- The study of disease producing parasites.

Pathology - The study of effect of disease on the structure and function of the body.

Pharmacology - The study of drugs, their properties, effects and use in the management of disease.

Endocrinology - The study of endocrine glands and their secretions.

Section- B

CHAPTER- 2

Musculo-Skeletal System

The musculo-skeletal system provides a shape and frame work for the body, protection to the internal organs & systems and brings movement of the body. It is made up of:

(a) Skeleton (b) Skeletal muscles.

The Skeleton

It is the bony frame work of the body, supporting and protecting the soft tissues and organs. It is built-up of from a series of bones, supplemented at places by cartilage.

Bones

It is one of the hardest connective tissue, which consists of calcium, phosphorus, matrix & bone cells.

The matrix of bone is solid & rigid as it is impregnated with calcium salts. The human body system consists of 206 bones of various sizes.

The bone tissues are of two types:

(i) Spongy Bone Tissue- Found in the ends of longbones, the vertebrae, the wrist , ankles and in skull bones.

(ii) Compact Bone Tissue- Found on the surface of all bones.

Types of Various Bones

(a) Long Bones- It has a shaft and two enlarged ends. e.g. Femur (Thigh bone), Humerus (Arm bone)

(b) Short Bones- They are small and compact bones. e.g. Carpel (Wrist bone), Tarsal (Ankle bone).

(c) Flat Bones- They are made up of two layers of compact bones alongwith in between a layer of sponzy bone e.g. Ribs, Skull bones.

(d) Irregular Bones- They have variable shapes & sizes. e.g. Vertebrae. There are thirty three irregular bones- 7 cervical vertebrae, 12 dorsal or thoracic vertebrae, 5 lumber vertebrae, 5 sacral vertebrae and 4 coccygeal vertebrae.

Structure of Bone

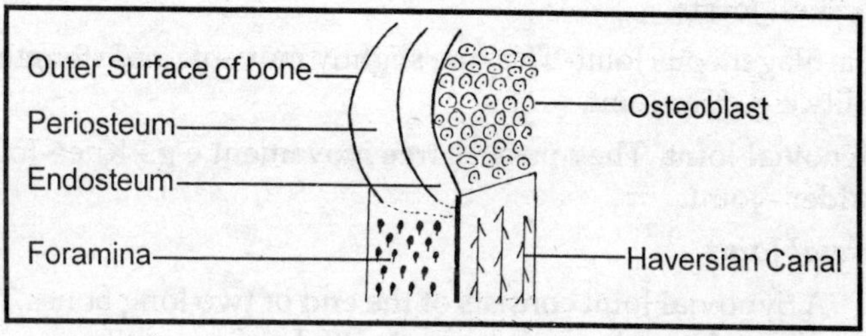

Fig.9

Bone consist of 50% solid and 50% water. Out of the 50% of solid their is 67% calcium salts and 33% cellular matter. The outer layer of bone is known as "Periosteum", the middle layer called "Endo-osteum" and the inner one area is known as " Osteoblastic", where the new bone cells are formed.

"Foramina" is a special type of stored food for the formation of bone cells and the "Haversian canal" is a tubular structure through which blood vessels and nerves passes to the bone tissue.

Protein is lay down in osteoblast and with the help of calcium,form bone cells which is known as"Osteoblast".The osteoblastic activities continue to take place regularly. The bone metabolism is known as "remoulding".

Cartilage

It is white,soft gelatinous special type of connective tissue,also can be considered as non-mineralised bone tissue.

Types of Cartilage

(a) Hyaline Cartilage- It is present at the end of bones forming a joint.It prevent frictions between the bone ends and allows smooth movement of the bones.

(b) White Fibro Cartilage- Found between the vertebrae and acts as a shock -absorber.

(c) Elastic Cartilage- It is flexible e.g.- the cartilage of the pina of the ear and larynx.

Joints

It is the meeting between two or more bones. Based on the structure, functions and purpose they are of three types

(a) Fibrous Joint- They are immovable and strengthen stability e.g. - Skull Joints.

(b) Cartilageneous Joint- They are slightly movable and stengthen stability e.g.-Hip-Joint.

(c) Synovial Joint- They possess free movement e.g.- Knee-Joint, Shoulder - Joint.

Synovial Joint

A Synovial Joint consists of the end of two long bones.The end surface of each bone is covered with hyaline cartilage.

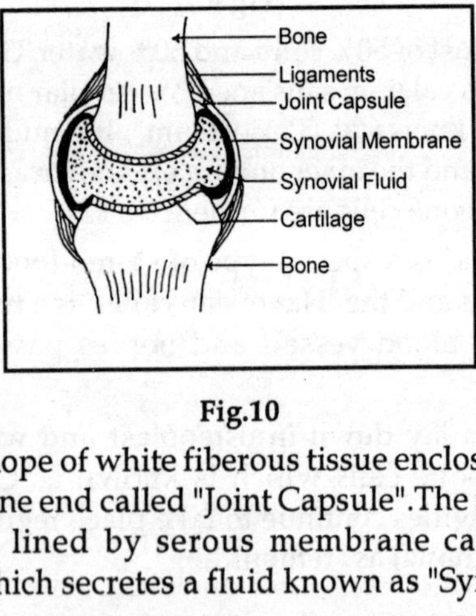

Fig.10

An envelope of white fiberous tissue encloses the joint and connects the bone end called "Joint Capsule".The inner surface of the capsule is lined by serous membrane called "Synovial Membrane", which secretes a fluid known as "Synovial Fluid".

The Synovial Fluid lubricates the end surface of bones and facilitates joint movements. Beside the capsule, thick strong bands of "ligaments" reinforce the joint outside the capsule.The muscles and tendons provides additional strength and stability to the joint.

Functions of the skeleton

(i) To serve as a structural frame work of the body.

(ii) To protect vital body organs and systems.

(iii) To act as levers,which is operated by the muscles, thus producing movements.

(iv) Bone serve as storage depot for calcium & phosphorus. 99 % of the total body calcium is stored in the bones and balance 1 % in the blood and tissues. The blood ionic calcium level is being maintained by the body through hormonal activities.

(v) The red bone marrow, which is present in the ends of long bones, ribs, etc., produces R.B.C.,W.B.C. and Platelets of the blood.

The Skeletal Muscles

As we know there are three types of muscles in the human body viz:

(a) Smooth or involuntary muscles,

(b) Cardiac muscles,

(c) Striated or voluntary or skeletal muscles.

The skeletal or striated or voluntary muscles are found in all parts of the body and can be moved at will, for example limbs, neck and trunk muscles.

It consists of long, mulltinucleated cells or fibres which show alternate dark & light bands across them.They are capable of quick, powerful and sustained contraction which are controlled by voluntary nervous system.

The muscles are enclosed in a fibrous sheath called the " Fascia", which at the end of bone becomes condensed to form cord called " tendon", that anchors the muscle ends to the bone.

The "bursa" is a sac like cavity filled with a viscid fluid and found in between tendon and bone, muscle and muscle, etc., and there by prevents friction between these surfaces.

The important skeletal muscles are deltoid (around the shoulder) and gluteus maximum (on hips),as they are relatively bulky and being used for intramuscular (I.M.) injection purpose.

The muscles are supplied with blood vessels,sensory or afferent and motor or efferent nerves for voluntary movements.

The skeletal muscles contain high percentage of protein. The regular exercise, protein rich diet & anabolic hormones promote its development.

Functions of the Skeletal Muscles

(i) To provide shape & size of the body

(ii) To bring about voluntary movements of various parts of the body.

Analgesic

The drugs which relieve pain are called analgesics. The analgesics act on the pain centre situated in the thalamus of the brain. The analgesic drugs are nonnarcotic or narcotic analgesics. Most of the analgesics belongs to the non - steroidal antiinflammatory drugs (NSAID) except narcotic analgesics and paracetamol and inhibit prostaglandin synthesis, thereby relieving inflammation and pain.

Antipyretic

The drugs which bring down elevated body temperature called antipyretic drugs. The antipyretic durgs act on the " heat regulating centre" situated in the hypothalamus and as a result brings about peripheral vasodilation and sweating, causing heat loss from the body.

The normal temperature varies from person to person between 97° F to 99° F. Commonly, by normal body temperature is meant 98.6° F (about 37° C).

Clinical Aspects

(a) Traumatic Disorders

Fracture- It means breaking of a bone. It may be simple or compound.The treatment of fracture involves reduction (Plaster) alongwith adequate supply of proteins, calcium and vitamins.

(b) Inflammatory Disorders

Arthritis- Inflammation of joints usually accompanied by severe & crippling pain and frequent changes in structure. It may be due to-infections (Pyogenic arthritis), injury (Traumatic arthritis), degenerative process (Osteo-arthritis), auto-immune response (Rheumatoid arthritis & Ankylosing Spondylitis), or metabolic disorder (Gout).

Arthralgia- Pain in the joint. The term used especially when there is no inflammation.

Bursitis- Inflammation of a bursa.

Fibrositis- Inflammation of non-articular white fibrous connective tissue with pain which affects soft tissue of the limbs & trunks. Cause is unknown.

Inflammation- It means reaction of the living tissue to injury, irritation, or infections.Symptoms are redness (Robor) swelling (Tumor), pain (Dolor), heat (Calor) and imparied functions of the affected part.

Prostaglandin and prostaglandin like substances are the main mediators of inflammation.

Lumbago- Pain in the lumber region (low back pain)

Myalgia- Pain in the muscles.

Myopathy- Any disease of the muscles.

Myositis- Inflammation of muscle, caused mainly due to viral infections, injection of highly irritant drugs. If extensive, may lead to necrosis, liquefacation, an abscess formation (Sterile abscess).

Osteoporosis- Thinning out of bone (loss of bone density) due to dranage of calcium & phosphorus from the bone, caused due to progressive loss of the protein matrix of the bone.

Osteomalacia- It is an adult form of rickets with softening and pain in the bone.

Osteomyelitis- Inflammation of bone, its covering membrane (Periosteum) & the bone marrow. Mostly caused by Staphylococci, Pneumococci bacteria.

Pain- It is an unpleasent sensation felt when impulses of noxious stimuli are transmitted to the brain through nerve fibres. The pain receptors are free nerve ending.

Rickets- It is a disorder of calcium & phosphorus metabolism associated with a deficiency of Vitamin - D. It occurs most often in infants and children up to 2 years.

Spondylitis- Inflammation of one or more vertebrae, without specific cause. It occurs mainly in young men.

Sprain- Injury to the soft tissues surrounding a joint (e.g.ligaments), resulting in swelling, pain & discoloration.

Teno-Synovitis- Inflammation of the thin synovial membrane of a tendon-sheath. It may be caused due to bacterial infection or mechanical irritation.

Tuberculosis of bone & joints- The tubercle bacilli settle in the bone usually near the epiphyseal cartilage where the synovial membrane is attached. Tuberculosis generally affects hip joint, knee joint and the spine. Treatment requires long term anti-tubercular drugs.

Applied Medicines

(i) *N.S.A.I.D's-* The non-steroidal anti-inflammatory drugs are those which exert their effect through inhibition of Prostaglandin synthesis. They provides analgesic, antipyretic (few of them) and anti-inflammatory effects (except dextropropoxyphine).

Aspirin-

Disprin (RCI), Colsprin (RCI), Micropyrin (Nicholas)

Ibuprofen-

Brufen(Knoll), Ibugesic (Cipla), Emflam (Merck), Ibuflamar (Indoco)

Diclofenac sod.-

Fensaide (Nicholas), Dicloran (Unique),Voveran (Novartis), Zobid (SG Pharma) Flexyl (Perch), Mobinac (Crosland), Jonac (Ger. rmedies), Diclonac (Lupin).

Diclofenac Pot.-

Votaflam (Novartis), Zix -50 (Jenburkt), Delta-K (Glat), Dolo-K (Mankind).

Piroxicam-

Brexic(Wockhardt), Dolonex (Pfizer), Movon-20 (IPCA), Pirox (Cipla)

Naproxen-

Artagen (Ranbaxy), Nalyxan (Lyka), Naprosyn (R.P.G.), Xenobid (Rallis)

Texoxicam-

Novotil (Recon), Tobitil (Ranbaxy)

Meloxicam-

M-Cam (Unichem), Melfalm (Cipla), Mel-Od (Zydus-Cadila)

Flurbirprofen-

Arflur (FDC), Flurofen (Hoechst), Froben (Knoll)

Indomethacin-

Idicin (IDPL),Indocap (Jagson Pal), Suract (SOL), Indoflam (Recon)

Mefenamic Acid-

Ponstan (Parke Davis), Meftal (Blue Cross), Lenagesic (Tata)

Ketoprofen-

Ketofen (PCI), Redufen (Unique)

Phenylbutazone-

Aristopyrin (Aristo), Kebutacine (Kee Pharma), Zolandin (SG Pharma)

Oxyphenbutazone-

Suganril (SG Pharma), Sioril (Albert David), Jagril (Jagson Pal)

Nimesulide-

Nimulid(Panacea), Nimid (Indoco),Nise(Dr.Reddy Lab.), Nimegesic (Alembic), Nimodol (Aristo), Nimuflam (J.K. Ph.), N-Lid Dt (Orchid), Nimuflex-Fd (Pharmed)

Auranofin(Gold)-

Goldar (Cadila H.C.), Ridaura (SB)

N.S.A.I.D'S. having proteolytic and mucolytic properties :

Chymotrypsin-

Chymoral (Elder), Alfapsin (Lyka),Soluzyme (lupin), Chymutrip (Bombay Tab.)

Serratiopeptidase-

Bidanzen (Glaxo-Welcome), Serazine (PCI), Emanzen (Emcure),

Seratio-M (Kee-Pharma),Seratid (Twilight), Biosuganril (S.G.), Tidase (Perch), Lyser (Comed), Primedase (Rallis)

Combination Drugs :

Serratiopeptidase+Diclofenac-

Seradic (Obsurge), Emangen-D (Emcure)

Diclofenac sod.+Paracetamol-

Diclogesic (Torrent), Dicloran-A (Unique), Esgipyrin (SG Pharma), Diclomol (Win-Medicare), Magadol (Alembic), Oxalgin-DP (Cadila H.C.), Parazobid (SG Pharma) Paranac (Twilight), Cofenac (Protec), Diclobid-P (Universal)

Ibuprofen + Paracetamol-

Bestophen(B.E.), Combiflam (Roussel),Ibugesic plus (Cipla), Emflam plus (Merck), Flexon (Aristo), Fenceta (Alkem), Ibuflamar P (Indoco), Neurophen (Ind-swift), Zupar (Allenburys), Imol (Recon), Dolomed (Comed)

Ibuprofen + Dextropropoxyphene-

Ibruvon Forte (Macleods) Lobain (DWD), Ibu-Proxivon (Wockhardt), Parvon Forte (Jagson Pal).

Paracetamol+Dextropropoxyphene-

Corbutyl (Roussel), Dexovon (USV), Dolapar Plus (Micro)

Propoxyphen + Paracetamol-

Sudhinol (Ranbaxy), Darvocet (Eli Lilly), Walagesic (Wallace)

Pentazocine+Paracetamol-

Expergesic (Win Medicare), Foracet (Ranbaxy)

Nimesulide+Paracetamol-

Dolamide (Ranbaxy), Sumo (Alkem)

(2) Muscle relaxants- They are centrally acting muscle - relaxants.

Baclofen-

Lioresal (Novartis)

Carisoprodol-

Carisoma & Carisoma compound (Wallace)

Chlormezanone-

Electrogesic (SOL), Powergesic (Jenbuerkt), Neurophen Compound (Ind-Swift)

Chlorzoxazone-

Duodil (Duphar), Flamar-P (Indoco),Parafon (Ethnor), Ibuflamar-MX (Indoco)

Methocarbamol-

Ibugesic-M (Cipla), Robiflam (Khandelwal), Flexinol (Protec)

Orphenadrine-

Orphamol (Torrent), Orphipal (Glaxo)

Tizanidine-

Sirdalud (Novartis), Tizan (Sun)

Valethamate-

Epidosin (TTK), Valosin (Sigma)

Besides, benzodiazepines (Diazepam, Chlordiazepoxide, etc.) acts as an effective skeletal muscle relaxants.

(3) Rubefacients & Topical Analgesics- The topical analgesics used in the wide variety of conditions like sprains, strains, low back pain, fibrositis, tennis- elbow, etc.

Creams-

Flamar (Indoco), Medicreme (Rallis), Multigesic (Nicholas) Muslax (B.E.), Zolandin (SG Pharma)

Ointments-

Relaxyl (Rallis), Dolopar (Micro), Sensur Rubefacient (Lyka)

Gels-

Dicloran Gel (Unique), Jonac Gel (German Remedies), Pirox gel (Cipla), Voveran Emulgel (Novartis), Tromagesic Gel (Themis Chem.), Fastum Gel (Menarini), Capsidol (Rexcel), Dolomed (Comed)

Spray-

Arjet Spray (Cadila)

(4) Other Drugs

Sulphasalazine-

Sazo-En (Wallace)

Glucosamine-

Cartilamine (Troikaa), Cartigen (Pharmed).

Section- B

CHAPTER- 3

Nervous System

The nervous system is made up of nervous tissue. Its function is to receive message or impulses from the environment and the body organs, to integrate & co-ordinate them and to send out messages to various organs and tissues,so as to bring forth an appropriate response.

Neurone

The nervous system consists of millions of nerve cells called "neurones",which communicate with one another at junctions called "synapses".

A synapse is formed between the axon of one neurone and either the cell body or dendrite of another neurone,which are not protoplasmically attached but separated by a tiny gap called"synaptic cleft."

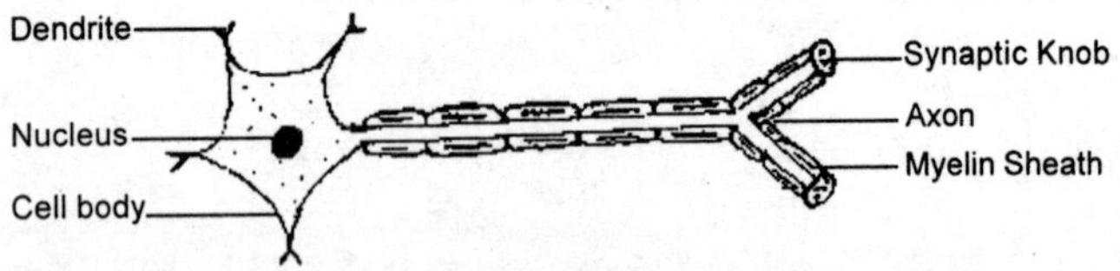

Structure of a Neuron

Fig.11

The junction between a muscle or a gland cell and an axon terminal is also a type of synapse called "neuro-effector junction". The neurone has got power of excitation and conduction.

The neurone cell membrane is polarised (electrically charged),becomes depolarised in response to a stimulus and thereby produces a tiny electrical current which is conducted (carried) along the neurone, either from dendrite to cell body or from cell body to axon.

When the impulse arrives at a synapse,it is transmitted to the next neurone.The conduction & transmission is brought about with the help of a chemical substance called a "transmitter", which is released from the terminal of axon and it combines with" receptors"on the dendrites or the cell body of the next neurone.

A number of chemical substances function as transmitters,viz.-Acetylcholine (Ach), Noradrenaline (NA), Serotonin and Dopamine.

An impulse is transmitted both across a synapse as well as across the neuro-effector junction.

Grey and White Matter

In the brain & spinal cord the area in which cell bodies of neurones are concentrated appears greyish in colour,called "grey matter ".And the area which is filled with nerve fibres i.e. axons & dendrites, appears white in colour, called "white matter."

In the brain grey matter forms a distinct layer at the surface known as "cerebral cortex", where as in the spinal cord grey matter is located around the centre.The grey matter are also found in the core of brain & the brain stem e.g.-basal ganglia,vagal nucleus, & vasomotor centre.

The white matter nerve fibres are collected into a clearly perceptible band known as " tracts" e.g. pyramidal tract & the spino thalamic tract.

Sensory or Afferent Nerve Fibres

The nerve fibres which carry impulses from the body organs to the central nervous system (CNS) called sensory or afferent nerve fibres.

Motor or Efferent Nerve Fibres

The nerve fibres which carry impulses from the CNS to the body organs, called motor or efferent nerve fibres.

Central Nervous System

It comprises of the brain and the spinal cord. The brain is situated in the skull and the spinal cord is enclosed with in the spinal canal and situated in tunnel passing through the vertebral column.

The brain and the spinal cord are covered by three membranes, the dura mater, the arachnoid mater & the pia mater and jointly called " Meninges". The dura mater & the arachnoid mater are in contact with the inner surface of the skull and the spinal cord. Whereas the pia mater closely envelopes the brain & the spinal cord.

Between the arachnoid & the pia mater there is a space known as the "sub-arachnoid space", which is filled with a fluid known as "cerebro-spinal fluid" (CSF).

The meninges are highly rich in blood vessels. The CSF is very much similar to tissue fluid and serves as cushion to the brain & the spinal cord against jerks or movements.

The CSF is produced by the network of blood vessels known as " choroidal plexuses", present in the cerebral ventricles.

The spinal cord ends at the level of first lumber vertebra of the vertebral column. Whereas the sub-arachnoid space extends upto the third lumber vertebra.

In the lumber puncture a needle is passed safely between IInd and IIIrd lumber vertebrae into the sub-arachnoid space for CSF examination, or for spinal anaesthesia or to inject drugs.

The Brain

The brain is divided in to three segments

(a) Forebrain or Cerebrum

(b) Midbrain

(c) Hindbrain.

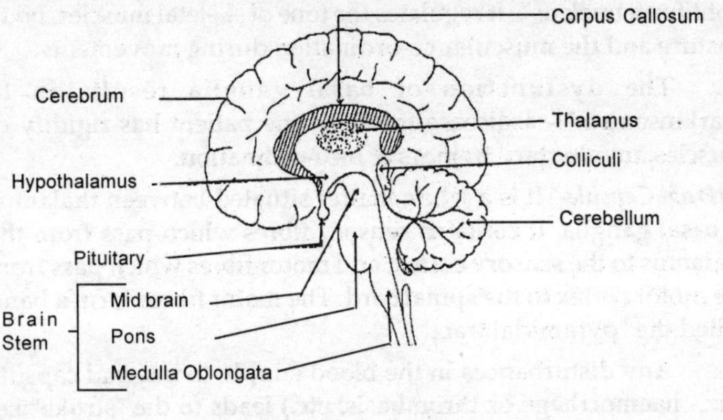

Sagital Section of the Brain (at midline)

Fig.12

(a) Forebrain or Cerebrum

It is made up of two hemispheres which are joined together with a thick band of nerve fibres, called " corpus callosum". Each hemisphere has a surface layer of grey matter known as " cortex" and a core of white matter containing sensory and motor nerve fibres.

Each cerebral hemisphere is divided into four lobes

(i) Frontal Lobe- It consist of higher function area which is concerned with memory, intelligence and thinking. Motor area controls the voluntary movements of the opposite half of the body and the speech area concerned with speech.

(ii) Parietal Lobe- It lies behind the frontal lobe and separated by central sulcus. It has sensory area & receives message from the opposite half of the body at the conscious level.

(iii) Occipital Lobe- Situated at the rear end of the cerebral hemisphere & concerned with the function of sight (Eye).

(iv) Temporal Lobe- It contain hearing area and area for the sensation of smell and for the regulation of emotions.

Thalamus- It lies close to the third ventricle and in the core of each cerebral hemisphere, in a large mass of grey matter. It receives sensory impulses from the opposite half of the body.

Basal Ganglia- These includes the "candate nucleus" and the "lontiform nucleus" . It regulates the tone of skeletal muscles, body posture and the muscular co-ordination during movements.

The dysfunction of basal ganglia results in to "parkinsonism" - a disease in which the patient has rigidity of muscles, involuntary tremors & inco-ordination.

Internal Capsule- It is a white matter situated between thalamus & basal ganglia. It contains sensory fibres which pass from the thalamus to the sensory cortex, and motor fibres which pass from the motor cortex to the spinal cord. The motor fibres form a band called the "pyramidal tract".

Any disturbances in the blood supply to internal capsule (viz.- haemorrhage or thrombosis, etc.) leads to the "stroke" i.e. paralysis of the other half of the body.

Hypothalamus- It lies in the floor of the third ventricle as a mass of grey matter and contains centres which control autonomic nervous system (control of vital functions such as respiration, metabolism & circulation).

The hypothalamus also provides some hormones which are carried out to pituitary gland situated just below it. So indirectly hypothalamus controls endocrine glands.

(b) Mid Brain

It is a short, thick stalk lies in between the cerebrum and the pons. The central canal of the mid brain connects the third and the fourth ventricles.

The anterior portion of the mid brain has the sensory fibres, the motor fibres, centres for co-ordinating muscular movements & for eye movements.

The posterior portion of the mid brain has four colliculi (a swollen structure), the upper two work as the relay station for visual impulses and the lower two for hearing impulses in the reflex arcs of visual and auditory reflexes.

(c) Hind brain

The hind brain consists of the "pons", the "cerebellum" and the "medulla oblongata".

Pons- It is situated inbetween the mid brain & the medulla oblongata and connects the two halves of the cerebellum with each other and with other parts.

The sensory and motor fibres passed through it and the nuclei from which 5th, 6th and 7th cranial nerves arise are also located in it.

Cerebellum

It is situated behind the pons and medulla and below the posterior end of the cerebrum. It is concerned with muscular co-ordination, maintenance of balance and regulation of posture.

Medulla Oblongata

It connects the pons with the spinal cord. The mid brain, pons and medulla oblongata together form the "brain stem".

The collection of grey matter which is distributed diffusely between the interlacing fibres of the brain stem, is called "reticular formation" (RF) and is concerned with the regulation of sensory impulses, learning and consciousness.

The medullary R.F. contains the vasomotor centre to control the heart & circulation, the respiratory centre, the vomiting centre and the chemoreceptor trigger zone (CTZ), which initiates vomiting when stimulated by chemicals circulating in the blood.

The medulla also contains nuclei for last five (8th to 12 th) cranial nerves.

Cranial Nerves

There are 12 pairs of the cranial nerves, out of which 3 are sensory, 5 are motor and 4 are mixed. They arise from the brain and form a part of the peripheral nervous system.

Spinal Cord

The spinal cord extends from the base of skull to the Ist lumber vertebra of the spine. The central canal of the spinal cord is surrounded by grey matter. The grey matter have three projections or horns on either side, known as "Anterior", "Posterior" and "Lateral horns".

The white matter of the spinal cord contains ascending and desending tracts of nerve fibres. e.g. - spino-cerebellar tract, spino-thalamic tract, etc.

The spinal cord gives rise to 31 pairs of spinal nerves. Of the 31 pairs of spinal nerves 8 are cervical, 12 are thoracic, 5 are lumber and 6 are sacral spinal nerves. Each nerve arising from the spinal cord has two roots-anterior and posterior.

Reflex Action

The communication of the nervous system is based upon the "reflex action" which communicates via a receptor organ, a sensory neurone, a connector neurone, a motor neurone and a effector organ. This chain is called as "reflex arc".

The reflex action involves:

(i) Reception of a sensory impulse

(ii) Its transmission to a motor neurone by means of one or more connector neurones.

(iii) Issuing of a motor impulse to the effector organ.

The reflex actions may be either facilitated or inhibited by modifying influences, either conscious or unconscious, from various areas of the central nervous system.

Autonomic Nervous System

The autonomic nervous system regulate the function of viscera or internal organs viz. - Lungs, Heart, Digestive tract, etc.

It is also known as visceral or vegetative or involuntary nervous system. The autonomic nervous system consist of two division - "Sympathetic" and "Parasympathetic".

Each organ is provided with a sympathetic and a parasympathetic nerve supply and its functional state at any one moment depends on a balance of the activities of the two nerves. The autonomic nervous system contains sensory and motor fibres too.

Sympathetic

It evokes a response from the organ appropriate for a stress situation. The motor sympathetic nerve fibres arise from neurons in the lateral horns of the thoracic and lumber segments of the spinal cord. The sensory sympathetic nerves run along with somatic sensory fibres in the posterior spinal cord.

Parasympathetic

It evokes a response appropriate to rest. The motor fibres of the parasympathetic system arise in the nuclei of the 3rd, 7th, 9th, and 10th cranial nerves, and in the lateral horn cells of the sacral segment of the spinal cord. The sensory parasympathetic fibres in cranial nerves have their cell bodies in the respective nuclei.

Both sympathetic and parasympathetic fibres have preganglionic fibres and postganglionic fibres.

All the preganglionic fibres of both parasympathetic and sympathetic are "cholinergic". When stimulated, release "acetylcholine" (Ach), and the drug which block the Ach receptor on ganglion called "ganglion-blocking drugs".

The postganglionic fibres are of two types:

(i) Adrenergic- They release "noradrenaline" (NA) when stimulated. They are sympathetic fibres (except of sweat glands)

(ii) Cholinergic- They release "acetylcholine" (Ach) when stimulated. They are parasympathetic fibres as well as sympathetic fibres of sweat glands.

The drug which blocks the action of the NA or Ach chemicals called "adrenergic receptor blocking drugs" or "Cholinergic receptor blocking drugs", as the case may be. After the function is over, the transmitter are distroyed by following enzymes.

(i) NA by - Catechol - o - methyl transferase (COMT)

(ii) Ach by - Cholinesterase (ChE)

Adrenergic Receptor

They are of two types Alpha and Beta. The drugs which block them are known as "Alpha blockers" and "Beta - blockers" respectively.

Cholinergic Receptor

They are found in autonomic ganglia, in the skeletal muscles and in organs receiving post ganglionic cholinergic fibres.The drug which blocks the receptor in

(i) Ganglia - called "ganglion blocking drugs"

(ii) Skeletal muscles - called "neuromuscular blocking drugs".

(iii) Internal organs - called "anticholinergic drugs.

Higher Control

The lateral horn cells and the cranial nerve nuclei from which autonomic nerve fibres arise are controlled by impulses they receive from the hypothalamus, which in turn is influenced by impulses from the higher centres of the cerebrum.

That is why mental activities and emotions have remarkable effect on blood pressure, respiration, heart rate and gastro-intestinal functions.

The drugs which blocks alpha ,or beta,or cholinergic receptors, counters the effect of nerve stimulation.

Clinical Aspects

Anaesthesia- It is loss of sensation with loss of consciousness.

Anxiety- Feelings of fear, apprehension and dred.

Delirium Tremens- It is an abnormal mental conditions resulting from alcohol intoxication. The symptoms are terror, restlessness, hallucination & confusion.

Depression- It is an emotional disorder of two types-"reactive depression" (Neurotic type) occurs as a reaction to stress, "endogenous depression" (Psychotic type) arises spontaneously in the mind. In both the types the symptoms are almost same,viz.loss of intrest, feeling that life is not worth living , emotionalism and suicidal thoughts,etc.

Epilepsy- It is a disordered electrical activity of the brain.The 'fit' is caused with loss of consciousness.

Encephalitis- It is the inflammation of the brain.

Encephalomyelitis- The inflammation of the brain & spinal cord.

Hypothermia- The condition of below normal body temperature.

Insomnia- A condition of sleeplessness.

Meningitis- The inflammation of the meninges.

Migraine- A unilateral periodic throbbing headache associated with nausea or vomiting and photophobia.

Neuralgia- The pain in the distribution of a nerve.

Neuritis- It is an inflammation of a nerve.

Neurapraxia- The temporary loss of functions in peripheral nerve fibres, commonly due to prolonged pressure or crushing.

Neurosis- It is a psychogenic disorder arises as a result of stresses and anxieties in the patient's enviornment.

Palsy-It is a facial hemiparesis of unknown cause resulting from oedema of the seventh cranial nerve.

Pain- It is an unpleasent sensation felt when impulses of noxious stimuli are trasmitted to the brain through nerve fibres.The pain receptors are free nerve ending.

Paralysis- A complete or incomplete loss of nervous function to a part of the body. This may be sensory or motor or both.

Pyrexia- The elevation of body temperature above normal(fever).

Parkinsonism- It is a syndrome of mask-like expression, tremor of the limbs, shuffling gait, pill rolling movements of the fingers.It can be of drug induced, post encephalitic, degenerative or arteriosclerotic.

Psychosis- It is a mental illness arising in the mind itself.

Schizophrenia- A group of mental illness characterized by disorganiza tion of the patient's personality which is often a lifelong illness. Common in youth or early adult life and its onset is sudden or insidious. Its symptom in childhood is called "autism".

Tremor- It is an involuntary trembling.

Thyrotoxicosis- It is an autoimmune thyroid disease caused due to excessive production of thyroxine hormone. The symptoms are anxiety, tachycardia, tremor, sweating and increased appetite with weight loss.

Vertigo- It means giddiness,dizziness.

Applied Medicines

(1) Non-Opioid Analgesics

Aspirin-

Apidin(IDPL), Disprin (RCI), Micropyrin (Nicholas)

Paracetamol-

Crocin(SB), Calpol (Wellcome), Metacin (Themis Pharma), Febrinil (Sigma), Pacimol (IPCA), Pyrigesic (East India)

Ketorolac-

Ketanov (Ranbaxy), Ketonic (Nicholas), Nato (Natco)

Propyphenazone-

Anafebrin (Themis Chem), Dart (Juggat)

Analgin-

Analgin (IDPL), Novalgin & Bralgan-M (Hoechst)

(2) Opioid Analgesics

Pentazocine -

Fortwin (Ranbaxy), Penzyl (Sigma), Pentawin (Biochem), Dolowin (B & B)

Propoxyphene & Dextropropoxyphene-

Sudhinol (Ranbaxy), Darvocet (Eli Lilly), Corbutyl (Roussel), Proxyvon (Wockhardt), Parvon (J.P.), Walagesic (Wallace), Centrivon (Macleods)

Morphine-

Morcontin continus (Modi-Mundi)

Ethoheptazine-

Equagesic (Wyeth)

Buprenorphine-

Norphin (Unichem), Pentorel (Khandelwal), Tidigesic (Sun), Glorphin (Glad)

Tramadol-

Contramal (SG Pharma), Tramazac (Cadila H.C.), Trasic (Kopran), Adamon (G. Remedies), Orchidol (Orchid)

(3) Anaesthetics- The drug which provides anaesthesia i.e. loss of consciousness. They are of three types, viz. - local, general and spinal anaesthesia.

Ketamine-

Ketmin (Themis Chem.), Ketalar (Parke Davis)

Lignocaine-

Gesicain (SG Pharma), Xylocard (Astra - IDL)

Bupivacaine-

Marcain (Sarabhai), Sensorcaine (Astra - IDL)

Thiopentone -

Intraval sodium (Rhone Poulenc), Anesthal (JP)

Halothane-

Fluothane (ICI)

Pancuronium Bromide-

Panconium (Khandelwal), Pavulon (Infar)

Vecuronium Bromide-

Norcuron (Infar)

(4) Hypnotics- A drug which produces a sleep resembling to natural sleep.

Nitrazepam-

Dormin (Micro), Hypnotex (PCI), Nitrosun (Sun)

Flurazepam-

Nindral (Torrent), Fluraz (B.B.)

Triclofos Sod-

Tricloryl (Glaxo), Pedicloryl (A. Remedies)

Zopiclone-

Zonap (Uniserch), Zopicone (Intas), Zopitran (Megacare), Zolinox (Solus)

*(5) Sedatives and Tranquilizers-*They produces anxiolytic, musclerelaxant, hypnosedative and anticonvulsent actions.

Chlordiazepoxide-

Equilibrium (Jagson Pal), Librium (Piramal H.C.) Equirex (JP), Libotrip (Merind)

Diazepam-

Anxol (Sigma), Calmpose (Ranbaxy), Paxum (East India), Valium (Piramal H.C.), Placidox (Lupin)

Lorazepam-

Ativan (Wyeth), Calmese (Themis Chem.), Larpose (Cipla).

Hydroxyzine-

Atarax (Uni-UCB)

Buspirone-

Anxipar (Torrent), Buscalm (Merind), Buson (Korpan)

Alpruzolam-

Alprax (Torrent), Alzolam (Sun), Trika (Uniserch), Zenax (DRL), Zolipax (Reliance), Anxit (Micro), Quite (Ind-Swift)

(6) Antipsychotics- They exerts its specific effect upon the brain cells.

Haloperidol-

Depidol (Torrent), Halidol (Glaxo), Serenace (RPG), Relianase (Reliance)

Fluphenazine-

Anatensol (Sarabhai), Prolinate (Sun)

Pimozide-

Neurap (Torrent), Orap (Ethnor), Pimodac (Alidac)

Clozapine-

Lozapin (Torrent), Sizopin (Sun)

Trifluoperazine-

Trinicalm (Torrent), Neocalm(Intas), Relicam Forte (Reliance)

Penfluridol-

Flumap (Torrent), Penflur (Mejda),Semap (Ethnor)

Thioridazine-

Mellaril(Novartis), Ridazin(Sun),Thioril (Torrent)

Risperidone-

Respidon (Torrent), Rispid (Panacea), Sizodon (Sun)

(7) Antidepressants- The drug that reduces depression. It is required minimum 3-4 weeks atleast to get any anti-depressant effects. They block the neuronal uptake of noradrenaline and exert anticholinergic activity.

Imipramine-

Antidep (Torrent), Depsonil (SG Pharma) , Tancodep (Torrent), Diamin plus (Reliance), Deplam (Mankind)

Nitroxazepine-

Sintamil (Novartis)

Clomipramine-

Clofranil (Sun), Clomifril (Torrent)

Amitriptyline-

Amitrol (Torrent), Librotryp (Merind), Tryptomer (Merind)

Doxepin-

Doxetar (Torrent), Doxin (Intas), Spectra (Solus)

Dothiepin-

Prothiaden (Knoll), Exodep (Sun)

Fluoxetine-

Fludac (Cadila), Flufran (Unique), Oxedep (Torrent), Prodep (Sun), Noc (Mano), Nuzac (Protec)

Nortriptyline-

Sensival (Wallace), Primox (Sun)

Mianserin-

Tetradep (Torrent), Depnon (Infar)

Trimipramine-

Surmontil (Rhone-Poulenc)

Amineptine-

Survector (Serdia)

Sertraline-

Serlift (Solus), Serta (Unichem), Sertil (SPPL)

Trazodone-

Trazodep (Torrent),Tazodac (Alidac),Trazonil (Intas)

*(8) Antiepileptics/Anticonvulsants-*The drug which prevent or stop convulsions. The aim of the therapy is to prevent seizures by maintaining an effective plasma concentration of antiepileptic agents.

Phenobarbitone-

Gardenal (Rhone-Poulenc),Luminal (Bayar)

Carbamazepine-

Carbatol (Torrent), Mazetol (SG Pharma), Tegrital (Novartis), Mezapril (Reliance)

Phenytoin Sod-

Dilantin (Parke Davis), Eptoin (Knoll), Epsolin (Cadila H.C.), Epilan (AFD)

Clonazepam-

Lonazep (Sun), Rivotril (Pirmal H.C.), Epitril (Novartis)

Ethosuximide-

Zarontin (Parke Davis)

Gabapentin-

Neurontin (Parke Davis)

Sod. Valproate-

Epilex (Knoll),Valparin (Torrent), Valtril (Merind).

Primidone-

Mysoline (ICI)

Clobazam-

Frisium (Hoechst), Lobazam (Sun)

*(9) Rigidity and Tremor Controllers-*The aim of therapy is to correct this imbalance even though the progression of the disease is not halted.Used mainly in Parkinsonism.

Levodopa-

Bidopal (Glaxo), Levopa (Wallace)

Selegiline-

Jumex (Torrent), Selgin (Intas), Eldepryl (Themis CH.)

Trihexyphenidyl-

Hexinal (Torrent), Pacitane (Cyanamid), Parnon (Sigma), Triphen (Sun)

Piribedil-

Trivastall (Serdia)

Bromocriptine-

Proctinal (Glaxo), Criptal (Helios)

(10) Cerebral Activators- Drugs used mainly in symptoms & signs of cerebral aging, mental retardation in children and in cerebrovascular accidents.

Pyritinol-

Encephabol (Merck)

Piracetam-

Normabrain (Torrent), Piratam (Croydon), Nootropil (Uni-UCB), Neurocetam (B&B)

Nicergoline-

Sermion (Pharmacia)

(11) Antiemetics- Drug which prevents nausia and vomiting due to a variety of conditions.

Promethazine Theoclate-

Avomine (Rhone-Poulenc), Phena (Ind-Swift)

Trifluopromazine Hcl.-

Siquil (Sarabhai)

Prochlorperazine-

Stemetil (Rhone-Poulenc), Emidoxin (Rallis)

Dimenhydrinate-

Dramamine (RPG), Gravol (Wallace)

Metoclopramide-

Perinorm (IPCA), Reglan (CFL Pharma), Maxeron (Wallace)

Domperidone-

Domstal (Torrent), Domperon (Cadila), Endopace (Themis Pharma), Gastractiv (Ethnor), Normetic (Lupin), Stugil (Ethnor), Domperi (IPCA), Motinorm (Medley), Dom-Dt (Morepen)

Ondansetron-

Emeran (B.E.), Ondem (Alkem), Periset (IPCA), Vomiset (Indi Ph.), Osetron (D.R.L.)

Doxylamine-

Doxinate (Sigma), Doxila (Pure), Vomitex (Mankind)

(12) Drugs used in Migraine

Flunarizine-

Flunarin (FDC), Nomigraine (Torrent), Sibelium (Ethnor), Migon (Lesante)

Ergotamine-

Ergophen (Inga), Migril (Wellcome), Vasograin (Cadila)

Sumatriptan-

Migratan (Dabur), Sumitrex (Sun), Suminat (Natco)

Propranolol-

Inderal (ICI), Ciplar (Cipla), Betabloc (USV).

Section- B

CHAPTER- 4

Digestive System

The digestive system is designed for the ingestion of food, its digestion & absorption and elimination of the unabsorbed & indigestible residue.

It consist of several organs,viz.

(a) Mouth
(b) Oesophagus
(c) Stomach
(d) Small Intestine
(e) Large Intestine
(f) Liver & Gall bladder, and
(g) Pancreas

(a) Mouth

The "Mouth"comprises of the lips, tongue, oral cavity, palate, teeth and gums. The oral cavity at front is bounded by the lips,behind continued up to oesophagus,above it is coverd by the hard & the soft palates and on either side bounded by the cheeks.

The floor of oral cavity is formed by the tongue which is lined by stratified squamous epithelium,except its upper surface. The oral cavity is lined with stratified epithelium. The epithelium of both oral cavity & tongue is subjected to constant wear and tear. As a result for faster repair (rapid cell division) requires adequate supply of Vitamin B_{12}, Folic acid and other B-Complex factors.

The "teeth" of upper & lower jaws project into oral cavity and their roots in the jaw bones are coverd by fleshy gums.

Each one gets two sets of teeth,called "Milk teeth" or temporary teeth and "Permanent teeth".The milk teeth are 20 in numbers which begin to erupt between 6 months to 2 years of age, whereas the permanent teeth are 32 in number and begin replacing the milk teeth at about the six years of age . The permanent teeth continue to erupt up to 25 years of age & last teeth (Molar) is known as "Wisdom teeth."

Each tooth is made up of a "crown", a "neck"and one or more "roots". The surface of the crown is formed of "enamel", which is rich in calcium. The dentine is situated under the enamel and unlike enamel is very sensitive to the temperature & touch. At the core of the tooth is "pulp", which contains the sensory nerve fibre & blood vessels. The gums which cover the sides upto the neck of teeth are made up of spongy connective tissue.

The "tongue" is the organ of taste, also acts as an important part of speech mechanism. The tongue aids the chewing and swallowing of food.

There are 3 pairs of "salivary glands" known as, Parotid, Sublingual and Submandibular, and they open into the oral cavity by means of fine channels or ducts and secrete fluid called "Saliva."

In the mouth,the food is masticated into fine particles by the teeth and the tongue helps to turn & roll the food. The saliva contains an enzyme called "Ptyalin" which breaks down the cooked starch (Polysaccharides) into maltose (Disaccharides), also it acts as a lubricant and initiates the digestion of carbohydrates.

The secretion of saliva is a reflex action and is brought about by the sight or smell of food or by its taste. The food when is properly chewed or masticated into soft bolus, the tongue pushes it to oropharynx area, where the muscles of larynx are pulled towards upward direction so that the glottis closes against epi-glottis and the bolus of food slides over it into oesophagus

(b) Oesophagus or Gullet

It is a muscular tube, about 25 cm. long which begins at the lower end of pharynx and ends at the stomach. The opening of the oesophagus in to the stomach is guarded by a sphincter, called "Cardiac sphincter",which prevents the back flow of gastric contents into the oesophagus. The food passes from oesophagus by distention and contraction of its muscular wall to the stomach.

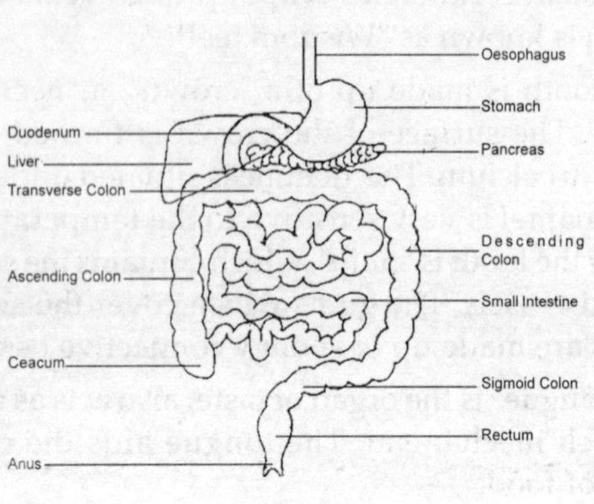

The digestive system.

Fig.13

(C) Stomach

It is a expanded 'J' shaped portion of the digestive tract.The stomach can be divided into three parts-"Fundus", "Body" and "Pyloric antrum".

The stomach at above opens in oesophagus and guarded by a muscular ring shaped sphincter called "cardiac sphincter", and below opens into "duodenum" & guarded by a sphincter called "pyloric sphincter".

The stomach wall like other walls of G.I.tract , consists of four layers,viz.-serous,muscular, submucosa and gastric mucosa epithelium.

The fundus gastric epithelium contains simple tubular glands, which secrete "mucus". The body gastric epithelium contains few "mucus secreting cells", "chief cells"-which secrete enzymes pepsin & renin and "parietal cells"-which secrete Hcl. The pyloric antrum contains "antral cells" -which produce a chemical messanger (hormone) called "gastrin".

The stomach recieves sensory nerve fibres through vagus and sympathetic nerves,the motor nerve fibres through vagus nerves. They stimulate contraction of stomach,secretion of Hcl & enzymes from the gastric glands. The motor nerve fibres are cholinergic and release acetylcholine (Ach).

The stomach performs the functions of digestion,

absorption, and a reservoir of food. The Hcl makes the gastric secretion acidic and lower the pH(below 4) thereby facilitating the action of "pepsin". The pepsin is an enzyme secreted by the chief cell, it breaksdown proteins into simpler units called "peptones".

The other enzyme, "renin" acts upon the milk & separates its protein, so that pepsin may act on it. If the pH of stomach rises due to lack of secretion or due to ingestion of an antacid, the action of pepsin is considerably diminished or inhibited.

The Hcl also acts as an antiseptic and kills bacteria or protozoa if any swallowed with the food . The secretion of Hcl in the stomach is stimulated by vagal stimulation, gastrin and histamine. The pyloric antrum produces a hormone called "gastrin", which stimulate Hcl secretion and an "intrinsic factor", which is essential for the absorption of Vitamin B_{12} from the duodenum.

The stomach normally takes about 3 hours to complete its digestive function and empty the contents into the duodenum, but it depends upon the type of meal, viz.-liquid, semi liquid, rich in fats, etc.

(d) Small Intestine

The small intestine comprises of three parts the "Duodenum", the "Jejunum" and the "ileum".The total length of small intestine is about 6.5 meters.

The duodenum is looked like 'C' shape letter. The Bile duct & the Pancreatic duct open into it by means of a common opening,through which the bile (bile acids and bile salts) and the pancreatic juice (Trypsin,Amylase & lipase enzymes) are poured in to the duodenum.

The duodenal mucosa secretes alkaline mucus to neutrilize acidic medium of the food flowing from the stomach. In duodenum the breakdown of protein (Peptone) to peptides, starch to maltose and fats into fatty acids & glycerol takes place with the help of pancreatic juice (See Table No.1).

The mucus membrane of the jejunum & ileum contains tubular glands called "crypts", which secrete erepsin, maltase, lactase and sucrase enzymes. It also have finger like projections called "villi", which increase the surface area for the absorption of digested food.

Organ	Digestive Fluid	Medium	Enzyme	Chemical Action/Job Function of an enzyme.
Mouth	Saliva	Alkaline	Ptyalin	Converts - Cooked starch to soluble Sugar (Maltose)
Stomach	Gastric Juice	Acidic	Pepsin Renin Lipase	Protein to polypeptide (Peptone) Milk Protein to casein Hydrolysis the fats
Duodenum	Bile	Alkaline	Bile	Emulsification of the fats
	Pancreatic	Alkaline Juice	Trypsin Amylase Lipase	Peptones to peptides All left over sugar to maltose Fats to glycerol & fatty acids
Small Intestine	Succus Entericus	Alkaline	Enterok-inase	Trypsinogen into active Trypsin & helps it to move further to the duodenum
			Erepsin	Reduces all left over poly-peptides to aminc acids
			Sucrase Maltase Lactase	Reduces all left over carbohydrates in to mono-saccharides, glucose, gla-ctose and levulose

Table No. 1 (The digestive enzymes & their functions)

The food is propelled along the small intestine by periodic waves of contraction called "Peristalsis."

The peristalsis is increased by vagal stimulation and diminished by sympathetic stimulation. The large number of micro-organisms live in small intestine as commensals, viz-E-coli, Bacteriodes, etc., some of these synthesize Vitamins (Niacin, Vit.-K).

(e) Large Intestine

The large intestine is about 1.5 meters long. It comprises of the "Caecum", the "Colon", the "Rectum" and the "Anal canal".

The main function of large intestine is to store and eliminate the undigested cr unabsorbed food residue.

The caecum is a bulb like portion of large intestine. Just below the ileum-caecum junction, there is a finger like projection called "Appendix", which opens into the caecum.

The colon consists of an "Ascending colon", a "Transverse colon", a "Descending colon", and a "Sigmoid colon". The sigmoid colon opens into the outside through rectum and anal canal. The anal opening is guarded by a ring of muscular tissue called "Anal sphincter".

At the large intestine water is absorbed along with glucose & sodium chloride,thus it help to regulate the fluid balance of the body.

(f) Liver and Gall Bladder

Liver is the largest gland in the body. It is known as metabolic workshop. The liver is situated below the diaphragm, in the upperpart of the abdominal cavity. Its weight is about 1.4 kg.,and consisting of two lobes, a right lobe and a left lobe.

The right lobe is larger than left lobe and situated in right hypochondrium. The left lobe is situated into epigastrium.

On the lower surface of the liver there is a cleft called "Porta hepatis", through which the portal vein & hepatic artery enter and the common bile duct & hepatic vein leave the liver.

Microscopically,the liver consists of hexagonal structural units called "Lobules",which at the centre has a vein called "Central vein" and alongside it has a bile duct and a lymphatic vessel. The liver cells are arranged around the central vein like the spokes of a wheel.

Each row of liver cells has a capillary or "Sinusoid" on oneside and a "Bile canaliculus" on the other. At the periphery of each lobule, a branch of hepatic artery and a branch of the portral vein opens together into the sinusoid, where the mixed blood then flows towards the central vein.

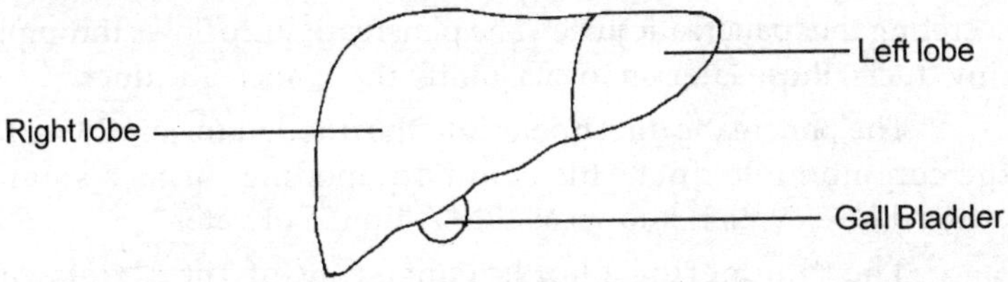

The liver(Front view)

Fig.14

The "Gall bladder ' is an oval fibro-muscular sac situated on the lower surface of the liver.It opens into "Cystic duct", which joins the common hepatic duct forming a "common bile duct."

The bile secreted by the liver is stored in the gall bladder. The bile contains bile pigments mainly "Bilirubin," and bile salts, viz-sodium glycocholate and sodium taurocholate.

The bile facilitates absorption of the fat soluble vitamins (Vit.A, D, E, K,), emulsification of the fats and their digestion and subsequent absorption.

The liver plays an important role in the metabolism of carbohydrates, fats and proteins .It also acts as an organ of storage for certain food stuffs.

The liver brings about chemical transformation of the foreign chemical substances including drugs and rendering them less toxic or nontoxic, more water soluble, thus facilitating their elimination through kidneys.

The glucose is converted into "Glycogen" by the process called "Glycogenesis and when needed, it is broken into glucose by the process known as "glycogenolysis".The glycogen is stored as food in the liver. The fat- soluble vitamins A, D, & K are stored in the liver, water soluble vitamins are not stored, execept a small quantity of Vit.-B_{12}.

(g) Pancreas

The pancreas is an elongated structure which is broad at one end and tapering at the other end.It is about 12-15 cm. long, situated horizantly below & behind the stomach.

The pencreas is a mixed gland, it contains "Exocrine glands" secreting the "pancreatic juice".The pancreatic juice flows through tiny ducts, those later on forms jointly the "Pancreatic duct."

The pancreatic duct opens into the duodenum jointly with the common bile duct.This common opening forms a small crater-like elevation known as the "Ampulla of vater."

The "Endocrine glands"consisting of the "Islets of langerhans" and secrete two hormones,viz- "Insulin" and "Glucagon."

The pancreatic juice contains enzymes, viz-trypsin, amylase and lipase, which digest proteins, carbohydrates and fats respectively.

Clinical Aspects

Achlorhydria- Absence of Hcl in the stomach, as found in the perniciousanaemia.

Anal fissure- A linear ulcer on the margin of the anus.

Anorexia- Loss of appetite for food.

Caries- It is the destruction of the tooth enamel.

Cheilitis- Inflammation of the lips.

Cheiolosis- Maceration at angles of Mouth.

Cholaemia- The presence of bile in the blood.

Cholangitis- Inflammation of the bile ducts.

Cholelithiasis- Formation or presence of gall stones in the gall bladder or bile ducts.

Cholecystitis- Inflammation of the gall bladder.

Cholera- An acute epidemic disease, in which evacuation of copious'Rice water' stools accompained by agonizing cramps. It is caused by "Vibro-comma."

Cholestasis- Diminution or arrest of the flow of bile.

Colic- Severe pain resulting from periodic spasm in an abdominal organ.

Colitis- Inflammation of colon, caused by worms or micro-organism.

Constipation- It is usually delay in the emptying of the colon.

Dental Abscess- The infection at the root of a tooth, mainly caused by pus producing bacteria (Streptococci, Staphylococci).

Diarrhoea- Deviation of bowel rhythm characterised by frequent and loose motions.

Dysentery- Painful loose motion accompanied by passage of mucus & blood in the stools.

Dyspepsia- It means indigestion.

Enteric fever- An infectious disease caused by Salmonella typhi (Typhoidbacilli), involving the small intestine.

Enteritis- Inflammation of the small intestine, caused by irritant or infection.

Flatulence- Gastric & intestinal distension with gas.

Gastritis- Inflammation of the stomach.

Gingivits- Inflammation of the gums.

Glossitis- Inflammation of the tongue.

Haemorrhoides- A condition in which a portion of the network of veins in the anal region proliferates, gets congested and forms a inflammed covering with mucus membrane. It may be a painful condition and can lead to anaemia due to chronic blood loss.

Hepatocirrhosis- A condition in which patches of liver cells are distroyed and replaced by fibrous tissue.

Hepatomegaly- Enlargement of the liver.

Hepatitis- Inflammation of the liver cells.

Hernia- The abnormal protrusion of an organ or part of an organ, through an aperture in the surrounding structure.

Hyperacidity- Excessive secretion of Hcl in the stomach.

Jaundice- It is a clinical term referring to the yellow appearance of the skin, & mucus membrane due to increase in bilirubin concentration. The main symptoms are dark urine, pale/clay coloured stool, anorexia, itching, weight loss, vitamins deficiency and pain in the joints.

Meteorism- Excessive accumulation of gas in the intestine.

Oesophagitis- Inflammation of the oesophagus.

Pancreatitis- Inflammation of the pancreas.

Pepticulcer- The ulcer occuring in the inner lining of the lower part of oesophagus, stomach and/or the first part of duodenum, when they are exposed to the action of pepsin in an acidic environment. (Gastric ulcer+Duodenal ulcer=Peptic ulcer)

Peritonitis- Inflammation of the peritonium.

Procititis- Inflammation of the rectum.

Proctalgia- The presence of pain in the rectal region.

Spasm- An involuntary muscular contraction.

Stomatitis- Inflammation of the buccal mucous membrane.

Vomiting- Forcible expulsion of gastric contents through the mouth.

Applied Medicines

(1) Antacids- They act locally, useful in the treatment of ulcer and non-ulcer dyspepsia. Almacarb(Glaxo), Digene gel(Knoll), Diovol (Wallace), Gelusil MPS (Parke Davis), Mucaine (Wyeth), pH_4 (B.E.), Polycrol Forte (Nicholas), Siloxogene (RPG), Ulgel (Dabur)

(2) *H_2 Receptor Antagonists*-They heal ulcer by blocking H_2 receptors.

Cimetidine-

Cimetiget (Franco), Ulciban (Torrent), Cimetidine(Cadila H.C.)

Ranitidine-

Aciloc (Cadila Ph.) Histac (Ranbaxy), Rantac (Unique), Ranitin (Torrent), Ulcitab (Themis Ph.), Zinetac (Glaxo).

Famotidine-

Blocacid (IPCA), Famocid (Sun), Famtac (Nicholas), Tobur (Themis Ph.), Topcid (Torrent), Zactane (Wyeth).

Roxatidine-

Rotane(Hoechst), Zorpex(Stancare)

(3) Colloidal Bismuth- They have cytoprotective and possible local prostaglandinstimulation properties. It also has a bactericidal action against Hellicobacter pylori (found in 90%of duodenal ulcer case).

Tripotassium dicitrato bismuthate- Denol (Elder), Pylocid (Merck), Trymo (Raptakos)

(4) Proton Pump Inhibitor- They inhibit gastric proton pump in the parietal cells there by reducing both basal & stimulated acid secretion.

Omeprazole- Ocid (Cadila H.C.),Omepral (FDC), Omez (DRL), Omezol (Alembic), Lomac (Cipla), Ulzol (Dabur)

Lansoprazole-

Lansofast (Cadila H.C.), Levant (Ranbaxy), Lanzap (DRL), Lanzol (Cipla), Lanzo (Indon)

Pantaprazole-

Pantocid (Sun), Pantodac (Alidac)

(5) Cytoprotectants- They provides an altrenative in reducing gastric acid by enchancing muscosal protection.

Sucralfate- Mecogard (Themis Ph.), Sucrase (Cadila-H), Ulcerfate (Sun), Sucramal (Menarini), Sparacid (A.Remedies)

(6) Prokinetic Agents- They restore gastric motility by indirectly enhancing acetylcholine release from myenteric plexus. Useful in reflex oesophagitis.

Cisapride-

Cisawal (Wallace), Esorid (Sun), Nupride (East India), Motilax (USV), Ciza (Intas), Cisapid (Kopran), Cisanorm (Gufic), Santiza (Lesante), Syspride (Systopic), Pulsid (Max)

(7) Antispasmodics/Anticholinergic- They inhibits parasympathetic innervation and thereby reduces secretion and motility of the stomach & intestine and relieve spasm of smooth muscles.

Hyoscine Butyl Bromide-

Buscopan(German Remedies).

Propantheline Bromide-

Pepler (Sun), Probanthine (Searle).

Oxyphenonium Bromide-

Antrenyl (Novartis), Alupromate (Remedies-I), Ulpane (Syno-Kem)

Mebeverine-

Colospa (Duphar).

Clidinium Bromide-

Equirex (Jagson Pal), Librax (Piramal H.C.), Spasril(Solus)

Isopropamide-

Gastabid(Torrent), Stelbid (SB).

Dicyclomine-

Colimex (Wallace), Cyclopam (Indoco), Dysmen (Sigma), Colinol (Noel), Neurospas (Ind-Swift), Spasmo-Proxyvon (Wockhardt), Synalgesic (Wyeth), Clomin (Core), Spasmindon (Indon)

(8) Laxatives- Drugs used to treat constipation, pre and post operative evacuation Agarol(Warner), Cremaffin (Knoll), Dulcolax (German Remedies), Julax (Rallis), Cellubril (Astra-IDL), Duphalac (Duphar)

(9) Antidiarrhoeals- The drugs being used for the symptomatic relief of diarrhoea or dysentery of amoebic, bacterial or mixed origin.

Metronidazole-

Flagyl (Rhone-Poulenc), Metrogyl (Unique), Aristogyl (Aristo)

Furazolidone-

Furoxone (SB), Fudone (Euphoric).

Diloxanide furoate-

Entamizole (Knoll), Eldazole (Elder), Zoa Forte (Merind).

Tinidazole-

Fasigyn (Pfizer), Tiniba (Cadila H.C.), Zoacide (Merind).

Secnidazole-

Secnil (Rhone-Poulenc), Senizo (B.E.), Tagera (Unichem).

Hydroxyquinolones-

Amicline (Franco), Enteroquinol (East India).

Diphenoxylate-

Lomofen and Lomotil (RPG), Diaratril (Alpine)

Loperamide-

Diarlop (Jagson Pal), Lopamide (Torrent), Ridol (Gufic).

Metronidazole + Nalidixic Acid-

Bacigyl (Aristo), Gramogyl (Stancare), Nalidys (B.E.), Qugyl-N (RPG)

Metronidazole +Furazolidone-

Dependal (SB), Dysfur-M (B.E.), Fumedil (Ethnor), Flagyl-F (Rhone-Poulenc), Metrogyl-F (Unique)

Tinidazole + Norfloxacin-

Diaba (Sun), Norazol (Ranbaxy), Norflox TZ (Cipla), Nodd (J.K. Ph.), Enteromac (Mac), Meganeg (Dabur)

Tinidazole + Ciprofloxacin-

Brakke (Franco), Cifran-CT (Ranbaxy), Ciplox TZ (Cipla), Gastrogyl (B.E.), Loxitin (Cachet), Oracip-TZ (Mercury)

(10) Pancreatics- Drugs used for replacement therapy in pancreatic insufficiency.

Pancreatin-

Digeplex-T (Rallis), Enzar Forte (Elder), Festal (Hoechst), Pankreoflat (Duphar), Serutan (TTK), Biopank (Kee Ph.).

(11) Hepatobiliary Preparations- Drugs used for liver cells disorders and to treat gall stones where surgery is inadvisable. Essentiale (Rhone-Poulenc), Hepamerz (Win Medicare), Livage (Aristo), Livotone (East India), Neurotop (Universal), Neo-Hepatex (B.E.), Udca (Duphar), Bio-Hep (Kee Ph.) Sorbiline (Franco Indian), Sorliv (Makers), Trisoliv (Medley)

(12) Enzymes & Carminative- They are soluble colloidal proteins produced by living cells and used for the management of anorexia, flatulence, dyspepsia, constipation, etc. Aristozyme (Aristo), Bestozyme (B.E.), Carmicide(Indoco), Dizytone (Unichem), Lupizyme (Lupin), Molzyme (FDC), Neopeptine (Raptakos), Pepfiz (Stancare), Unizyme (Unichem), Vitazyme (East India), Digeplex (Rallis), Vizylac (Unichem), Digestomen (Menarini), Genozyme (Geno), Merizyme (Mercury), Xymex (Medley)

(13) Drugs for fissure & Haemorrhoides- They are soothing preparations in the form of cream, ointments, suppositories, or foam applied locally to relieve pruritus ani or the pain of haemorrhoids. Anovate (Allenburys), Faktu (Crossland), Shield (SB), Proctosedyl (Roussel), Medithane (Weyth), Laxicon Enema (Stadmed), Mesacol Enema (Sun), Tab. Daflon (Serdia), Proctosedyl-M rectal cap (Roussel).

Section- B

CHAPTER- 5

Nutrition And Metabolism

The body is the product of its nutrition, as nutrition maintains life, growth, and normal functions of all cells & forming various tissues and organs. The nutrition of the body is largly dependent on the proximate principles. Following are the proximate principles:-

(1) Proteins

(2) Carbohydrates

(3) Lipids (Fats)

(4) Vitamins

(5) Minerals

(6) Water.

(1) Proteins

Proteins are the essential constituents of the protoplasm. Proteins are highly complex substances composed of large molecules containing Carbon (54%), Hydrogen (7%), Nitrogen (16%), Oxygen (22%), sometimes contain Sulphur, Phosphorous and other elements.

Proteins are made up of units called "Amino Acids" .The amino acids can be put together in a number of ways to form various proteins. Protein can be divided into:

(a) Simple Proteins (e.g. Albumin, Globulins, Scleoroproteins, Protamine.)

(b) Conjugated Proteins (e.g. Haemoglobin, DNA, RNA, Phosphoproteins, Lipoproteins.)

(C) Derived Proteins (e.g. Polypeptides, Peptones, Amino acids, etc.)

Sources of Proteins- There are two main sources of proteins

(a) Vegetables (e.g. Groundnut, Peas, Soyabeans, Pulses, Wheat, Rice.)

(b) Animals (e.g. Meats, Fish, Eggs, Milk & Milk products.)

Amino Acids- The amino acids are the basic units of proteins. They can be classified as

(a) Essential Amino- Acids- They cannot be synthesized in the human body & must be provided in the diet to meet the body's requirements. The eight essential amino-acids are:

Leucine, Isoleucine, Valine, Threonine, Lysine, Methionine, Tryptophan, and Phenylalanine.

The lack of one of the essential amino acids lead to a negative nitrogen balance, fatigue, loss of appetite & irritability. The health is restored when the missing amino acids are added in the diet.

(b) Non-Essential Amino-Acids- They are synthesized in the human body from the breakdown of proteins. The non-essential amino-acids are:--Histidine, Cystine, Tyrosine, Glycine, Arginine, Alanine, Cysteine, Glutamine, Aspargine, Serine, Proline, Hydroxy-Proline, Aspartic Acids & Glutamic Acid.

Proteins provide the basic material of every living cell viz., protoplasm . Protein is essential for repair & maintenance of tissues, and formation of new cells (growth in children, formation of foetus in pregnancy). Proteins are also necessary for the formation of Enzymes (Digestive Enzymes and all Enzymes involved in biological metabolism and functioning), Hormones (Growth Hormone, Oxytocin, Insulin, Vasopressin.) and Antibodies (Immunoglobulins responsible for immunity). Proteins act as buffers helping to maintain pH of the plasma, C.S.F., etc.

Protein also aids in the transport of nutrients (Lipoproteins) & drugs. They are also present in the human blood plasma and known as plasma proteins (viz. Albumin, Globulins & Fibrinogen). Since proteins are anabolic, so have little energy value. Protein provide 4 calories per gram.

(2) Carbohydrates

Carbohydrates are an organic compound containing carbon, hydrogen & oxygen. They are formed in nature by photosynthesis in the plants (except Lactose & Glycogen) & are heat producing viz. Starch, Sugars, Cellulose. Carbohydrates are classified in to three groups

(a) Monosaccharides (b) Disaccharides (c) Polysaccharides.

(a) Monosaccharides- They are simple sugars, which form the building blocks of other carbohydrates, e.g. Glucose, Fructose, Galactose.

(b) Disaccharides- They are compounds which can be split into two monosacchrides, e.g. Maltose, Lactose, Sucrose.

(c) Polysaccharides- They are complex & large carbohydrates e.g.- Starch, Glycogen.

The main function of carbohydrates is to provide fuel for the production of energy . They provide 4 calories per gram.

(3) Lipids (Fats)

Fats belong to a group of compounds called "lipids", which also include Phospholipids, & Sterols such as Cholesterol & Steroid hormone. Fats are esters of fatty acids and glycerol. They are of three types

(a) Simple lipids- Like Triglycerides

(b) Compound lipids- Like Phospholipids

(c) Associated lipids- Like Glycerol, Cholesterol, Steroid, Fattyacids.

There are two main sources of fats:

(i) Animal fats- Present in various Meats, Milk, Ghee, Cream, Butter, etc.

(ii) Vegetable fats- Present in Nuts, Olive Oil, Groundnut Oil, etc.

The difference between these two oils is the presence of high proportion of saturated fatty acids.

The main function of fats are to serve as source of energy for the body & to serve as a source of (especially animal fats) fat soluble vitamins. Fats provide app. 9 calories per gram.

(4) Vitamins

The vitamins are organic substances (mainly dietary constituents) required in small amount for the maintenance of health and growth. Thus vitamins are one of the essential substances for the life process. The vitamins are said to act like organic catalyst in various metabolic processes of the body. Most vitamins play a role of either enzyme or co-enzyme. There are 20 vitamins, five of them are produced in the body itself. Since all the vitamins are not synthesized in the body, therefore vitamins must by supplied in normal daily diet.

A "Recommended Dietary Allowance" (RDA) has been established for most of the vitamins in normal health conditions by the Nutrition Expert Group of the Indian Council of Medical Research.

Depending on their solubility, vitamins are divided into two main groups:

(a) Fat Soluble Vitamins

(b) Water Soluble Vitamins.

(a) Fat Soluble Vitamins

These are A, D, E, & K and are soluble in fats and absorbed in the presence of bile or pancreatic lipase. Normally these vitamins are stored in the liver. In case of excessive consumption, it can lead to vitaminosis.

(i) Vitamin-A- It is also known as "Retinol". It is present in the plants as beta-carotene, which animals & man can convert into retinol. The chief sources of vitamin-A are carrots, spinach, fish (cod & shark), liver, egg yolk, cream, butter and cheese.

The 0.6 mcg. of beta carotene is equivalent to 1I.U. or 0.3 mcg of retinol. The vitamin-A is measured in terms of international units (I.U.). The recommended daily in take is for the adults 2500 I.U. to 5000 I.U.

Functions

(1) Vitamin- A is an essential component of the "Visual purple" a photosensitive pigment present in the retina and helps the eye to function in the light that varies in intensity. Its deficiency causes night blindness, delayed dark adaptation & xeropthalmia.

(2) Vitamin- A is necessary for the normal health of the all epithelial membranes viz. skin, lining of eyes, intestines, lungs, etc. The deficiency of vitamin-A may decrease activities of the cells of immune system.

(3) Vitamin- A is necessary for normal growth, reproduction & immunity through out life. Its deficiency leads to retarded growth, dry & thickened skin, lining of respiratory tract & other passages.

(4) Vitamin-A (Beta-carotene specially) acts as an anti-oxidant. The anti-oxidant are the substances that protect against oxidative changes & damage caused by free radicals. These free radicals can damage DNA & other molecules. Oxidative damage has been implicated as a cause of ageing, cancer and atherosclerosis.

(ii) Vitamin-D- There are two important forms of Vitamin-D

(1) Cholecaliciferol (Vit-D_3) - The natural form synthesized in the skin in the presence of sunlight, thereby it is also known as sunshine vitamin.

The Vitamin D_3 is normally found in fish, eggs, milk and milk products.

(2) Ergocalciferol (Vit.-D_2)- It is rarely found in nature. It is synthesized from ergosterol found in the plants.

The Vitamin-D is also measured as I.U., one I.U. is equivalent to 0.025 mcg. of cholecalciferol. The recommended daily intake is 400 I.U. in children below 6 years and during pregnancy & lactation, 200 I.U. for adults.

Functions

It is necessary for the maintenance and growth of bones & teeth. Vitamin-D promotes absorption of calcium from the intestinal tract.

Its deficiency leads to rickets (bow legs) in the infants & children, osteomalacia (loss of calcium from bones) in adults.

(iii) Vitamin-E It is also known as "Tocopherol". Mainly found in wheat & rice germ oil, milk, green vegetables, eggyolk and soyabeans. The recommended daily intake is 10 to 30 mg. for adults.

Functions

(1) It promotes healthy circulatory system by preventing the formation of blood clots (atherosclerosis).

(2) It acts as an anti-oxidant (particularly on lipids) & protects RBC from damage by oxidation.

(3) It is desirable in fat metabolism syndrom, in premature infants on artificial foods & when large amount of unsaturated fatty acids are included in the diet.

(4) It eases osteoarthritic pain.

(5) It is also used clinically in the management or prevention of

repeated abortions, sterility, etc. though its role in these conditions is not established as the mechanism of action of Vit.-E is not fully understood.

Its deficiency may leads to haemolysis (rupture of RBC) and as a result anaemia.

(iv) Vitamin-K

It is found in green vegetable [spinach, peas], soyabeans & some tubers. In addition to natural dietary sources, it is also being produced by some bacteria in the small intestine.

Vitamin-K is absorbed from the intestine in association with dietary fats and requires bile salts to aid the emulsification and absorption of fats. A little part of Vit.-K is stored in the liver & the rest is utilized.

The usual recommened daily intake is 30 to 100mcg per day, depending on how much is being derived from intestinal synthesis by some bacteria.

Functions

It helps the blood clotting and its deficiency can occur owing to a number of causes and may lead to impairment of blood coagulation & haemorrhage. The prolonged use of antibiotic therapy may suppress the normal intestinal flora & reduce the synthesis of Vitamin-K.

(b) Water - Soluble Vitamins

These are the groups of Vitamins which include the Vitamins of B-complex and Vitamin-C. As they are water-soluble, they are not stored in the body. Therefore a constant & regular supply of these Vitamins in our diet is necessary. The deficiency of these Vitamins may lead to disease conditions and any excess being excreted in the urine

The B-Complex Vitamins are B_1(Thiamine), B_2(Riboflavin,), B_6 (Pyridoxin), B_{12} (Cyanocobalamin), Nicotinic acid, Pantothenic acid, Biotin & Folic acid.

(i) Vitamin B_1 or Thiamine

It is found in whole grains (not polished or milled grain, as it is present in the outer layer), meat, eggs, potatoes, nuts, pulses, and milk. The daily requirement is linked with the total carbohydrate intake. The average recommened daily intake is 1 to 2 mg. in adults.

Functions

It is used to release energy from carbohydrates & to transmit nerve impulses. Thiamine participates in the formation of co-carboxylase (co-enzyme in kreb's cycle), required for the decarboxylation of pyruvic acid and initiating its stepwise oxidation to CO_2 and water to yield energy. Thiamine is also needed for the synthesis of the neurotransmitter acetyl choline.

Its deficiency gives rise to the condition known as "beri-beri". The beri-beri is of two types wet beri-beri (referable to cardiovascular system) and dry beri-beri(referable to peripheral nerves). The symptoms in early stage are fatigue, lack of appetite, nervousness, depression, G.I. dysfunction, lassitude & irritability. In severe conditions it may lead to loss of muscle strength, oedema, enlargement of heart and peripheral neuritis.

(ii) Vitamin B_2 or Riboflavin

Vitamin B_2 or riboflavin found in milk, soyabeans, peas, liver and lentils. It is radily absorbed after being synthesized by bacteria of the normal intestinal flora. It occurs in nature as riboflavin, fiboflavin phosphate or flavoproteins. The flavoproteins play an important role in oxidative systems of living cells for the production of energy. The recommended daily allowance of Vitamin B_2 is between 1.5 to 2.5 mg.

Functions

It is well established that cellular growth can't occur in the absence of Vitamin-B_2 or riboflavin. Any local trauma to the skin (e.g. angles of the mouth, surgical incision, or other wounds) will be repaired by the local growth only to the extent that Vitamin-B_2 and protein are available . The cor nea being devoid of blood supply, needs adequate Vitamin-B_2 to carry on cellular oxidation.

Its dificiency gives rise to stomatitis, glossitis & conjuctivitis. The minor injuries become aggravated in Vitamin-B_2 dificiency as new cells can not grow to replace the damaged ones. The common symptoms are cracks appear at the corner of the mouth & the tongue become red & swollen. It is also found that in its deficiency R.B.C. have a shorter life span.

(iii) Vitamin-B_6 or Pyridoxine

The rich sources of Vitamin-B_6 are meat, liver, fish, yeast, milk, eggyolk, green leaves and whole grain cereals. The recommended daily intake of pyridoxine or Vitamin-B_6 is 2 to 3 mg. in adults.

Functions

It participates in enzyme systems concerned with protein metabolism. As part of the enzyme phosphorylase, it also facilitate the conversion of glycogen from liver & muscles into glucose phosphate thereby increases the stamina. Studies have shown that Vitamin-B_6 in high doses can prevent the build up of cholesterol in the blood and boost mental energy. Vitamin-B_6 plays an important part in the synthesization of haemoglobin. It also relieve the symptoms of premenstrual tension, acne, depression, breast pain & bloating.

The Vitamin-B_6 deficiency can lead to convulsions, irritability, failure to gain weight & hypochromic anaemia in infants. Alcohol, treatment with isoniazid, contraceptives and certain drugs used to treat hypertension may cause Vitamin-B_6 dificiency. The symptoms of Vitamin-B_6 deficiency include depression, headache & confusion.

(iv) Vitamin-B_{12} or Cyanocobalamin

It occours naturally in the foods of animal origin (Liver, Kidney, Meat, Fish) and in yeast. There are number of compounds which are closely related to cyanocobalamin & posses Vitamin-B_{12} activity, only one compound Hydroxocobalamin, is available for therapeutic use. They are (Cyanocobalamin & Hydroxocobalamin) bound more strongly to the serum proteins and excreted slowly by the kidneys. The recommended daily allowance of Vitamin-B_{12} is 1 to 2mcg. in adults.

Functions

Vitamin-B_{12} keeps our nerves in proper shape and along with folic acid is needed for the maturation of R.B.C. Vitamin-B_{12} or cyanocobalamin contains cobalt & is essential to the normal function of folic acid. Vitamin-B_{12} & folic acid participate in the intermediate stages of nucleic acid synthsis (DNA production).

Its deficiency gives rise to Pernicious Anaemia and a neurological syndrome known as "Subacute combined degeneration" of the spinal cord, this is a condition characterized by peripheral neuropathy and degeneration of the posterior and lateral columns of the spinal cord, having symptoms like numbness, pricky sensation in extremeties, burning feet, and delirium. Vitamin-B_{12}

deficiency may occur due to Alcohol consumption, Intestinal surgery, Medicines for the management or treatment of T.B., Hypertension, Gout & Parkinsons disease.

(v) Nicotinic Acid or Niacin or Nicotinamide

It is widely distributed in both animals and plants. The good source of Niacin are yeast, meat, liver, poultary, pulses, cheese, green vegetables, cereals and potatoes. It is synthesized by colonic bacteria & is absorbed from the intestine. The recommended daily intake of Niacin is 15 to 20 mg.

Functions

It is essential for cellular oxidation - reduction reactions & metabolism of carbohydrates, fats & proteins.

Its deficiency gives rise to a disease called Pellagra. Symptoms of this disease include diarrhoea, dermatitis, soreness of tongue & mouth, insomnia and mental confusion. Complete absence of Niacin in the diet for longer period may lead to psychotic disease called "Schizopherenia".

(vi) Pantothenic Acid

It is present in liver, eggs, yeast & whole grain cereals. It is present in most living cells as a constituent of co-enzyme -A. The recommended daily intake is set at 10 mgm, but is difficults to estimate accurately.

Functions

It is required for the synthesis of cholesterol & fatty acids, for the production of energy from fats, proteins & carbohydrates (at citric acid cycle). The pantothenic acid helps in the management of paralytic ileus, - a condition where peristaltic movements of the intestines are diminished or absent.

No definite symptoms of deficiency of this Vitamin have been established. The malnourished subjects may have burning feet syndrome, fatigue and the patient is listless.

(vii) Biotin

It is present in liver, eggyolk, nuts and legumes. Normal diet provides adequate quantity of Biotin.

Functions

Biotin plays a role in the formation of fatty acids and the metabolism of some amino-acids.

(viii) Folic Acid

It is widely distributed in nature. Found in green leafy vegetables, yeast, liver, mushrooms, nuts, pulses and floor & cereal food. Chemically it is pteroylglutamic acid (PGA). A number of analogues with PGA like activity are collectively reffered to as "Folates". Folates in the food are mainly present in conjugated form and are hydrolysed to folic acid and absorbed. Folic acid as such in not active, it is reduced in the body to dihydrofolic acid (DHF) & then to tetrahydrofolic acid (THF) or folinic acid - a co-enzyme of folic acid. The recommended daily allowance is 100 mcg. in adults & upto about 800 mcg. in pregnancy.

Functions

It is concerned with nucleic acid synthesis (DNA & RNA Synthesis), so folic acid is therefore necessary for cell division and maturation of erythrocytes [R.B.C's.].

Its deficiency gives rise to an anaemia called pernicious anaemia or megaloblastic anaemia. Folic acid deficiency has also been reported to be associated with neuropathy and spontaneous abortion. Its deficiency also leads to restless, depression.

(ix) Vitamin-C or Ascorbic Acid

It is present in citrus fruits, green leafy vegetables, and potatoes. The Ascorbic Acid defends us in tough situations from cold to cancer. The recommended daily allowance is 50 mg. in adults and 80 mg. during lactation.

Functions

It plays a role in the formation of intracellular cementing substance, fibrous tissue and collagen. If collagen is defective, the cells of the tissue are not bound properly together so that formation of tissues such as bone matrix, teeth, lining of blood vessels, gums etc. is impaired. Vitamin-C helps healing of wound & fractures. It also promotes iron absorption. Vitamin-C also acts as an antioxidant thereby protecting cells and delayed ageing.

Its severe deficiency gives rise to "Scurvy", characterised by pinpoint haemorrhage, spongy gums, weakness, slower wound healing & tenderness of legs. Smoking, alcohol consumption & oral contraceptives may leads to severe deficiency of Vit. - C.

(5) Minerals

Minerals are the foundation of health. They are as

important to health as vitamins .All vitamins do us little good without minerals. Our body contains a number of minerals. Some are present in very minute quantities known as " trace elements" and those present in larger quantities are known as "macro elements".

Trace Elements- Iodine, Copper, Manganese, Zinc, Cobalt, Selenium, Tin, Silicon, Chromium, Fluorine & Nickel.

Macro Elements- Sodium, Potassium, Calcium, Iron, Phosphorus, Magnesium & Sulphur.

The Calcium, Phosphorus & Magnesium are the constituent of bones & teeth. Many of the trace elements are concerned in the enzyme system in the body. Minerals which are soluble present inside the body cells are Potassium & Magnesium and outside the body cells are Sodium & Chloride. Minerals help us to cope with the specific problems of modern life such as stress and pollution. Zinc has been reported to shorten the convalscence period by improving wound healing. Minerals deficiency may leads to condition like hypertension, osteoporosis, anaemia, etc. So in other words , vitamins are important but minerals help to create total health.

A brief note on some important minerals is given below

(i) Sodium

We take sodium in our diet as sodium chloride. The daily dietary intake varies from 5 to 20 gm., low intake of sodium is advisable in certain diseases of kidney, heart and liver. Almost all the sodium intake is excerted through urine.

Its deficiency can occur in patients with low intake. The common symptoms are excessive sweating severe diarrhoea or vomiting and leads to a reduction in the volume of extracellular fluid and blood.

(ii) Potassium

All cells of animals & plants are rich in potassium. It can be obtained easily from a variety of foods particularly fruits & vegetables. Potassium is concerned with the regulation of fluid contents of the cell. It works as an electrolytes, and helps in nerves transmit message, there by ensures proper functioning of every muscle of the body, most notably of the heart muscles. Sudden drop in potassium (K) can cause cardiac problem. It was confirmed that ratio of sodium and potassium is 1:1 benificial for the normal human body.

Its deficiency can occur from increased loss due to vomiting, diarrhoea, continued use of diuretics and in wasting diseases. The common symptoms of 'K' deficiency are fatigue, tiredness, weakness , irritability and can be cardiac problem.

(iii) Calcium

Milk and some milk products such as cheese, yoghurt, small fish such as sardine, fruits and vegetables are good source of calcium. It is a bone saviour. Our cells need calcium to function properly. It blocks highblood pressure, inhibits cancer and fights cholesterol. It is absorbed in the small intestine in the presence of Vit-D. The recommended allowance for calcium for adults is 400 to 600 mg perday, children 800 mg.per day, and pregnancy & lactation from 1gm. to 1.5 gm. per day.

Calcium is essential for the formation of bones & teeth, for clotting and for normal functioning of nervous & muscular systems. Its deficiency is called hypocalcaemia, a condition where serum calcium level falls below 9 mg. per 100 ml. Its severe deficiency can lead to rickets in children and osteomalacia in adults. Loss of calcium after menopause leads to postmenopausal & senile osteoporosis. Hypocalcaemia can also lead to "tetany"-a condition of hyperexcitability of the nervous system caused by low calcium serum level or a change in the ratio of calcium to phosphorus in the serum. The common symptoms of calcium deficiency are cramps of skeletal muscles (hand & fingers, common in pregnancy), spasm of plain muscles of larynx, bronchi and G.I. tract. It can also produce uncontrollable temper and outburst, which usually occurs in a stressful condition.

(iv) Iron

Iron is the major component of blood . It is commonly found in most fruits and green vegetables. The iron dificiency is the most commonly encountered mineral deficiency in clinical practice especially in our country.

Iron deficiency leads to depletion of iron stores of the body. Anaemia may or maynot be present. The recommended daily intake of iron is 10 mg. for adults and 18mg. for women in child-bearing period. As usually consumed diet is barely enough to meet daily recommended intake in pregnancy and a large proportion of menstruating women, supplementation of iron is recommended in these susceptible groups. Iron absorption can be affected by acidic medium, presence of Vitamin- C & different iron forms (ferrous or ferric). Its deficiency may lead to anaemia.

(v) Phosphorus

It occurs in all living cells so it is found in most foods. Phosphorus like calcium is an essential constituent of bones and teeth. It is also needed in DNA & RNA formation. The energy produced by oxidation of glucose is stored in cells in high energy phosphate compound. Antacid affects its absoption.

Its dificiency does not occur in man because ample quantities are available through normal diet.

(vi) Magnesium

It is present in cereals, vegetables, dry fruits, soyabean,potatoes and oat meal. The recommended daily intake is 350 mg. to 450 mg. in adults. It work as an antioxidant.

It is an important intracellular mineral which plays an important part in many enzymatic reactions associated with neuromuscular contraction & protein synthesis. It is required for dilating the blood vessels, in lead poisoning. It also prevents & reverses diabetes. Small amount of magnesium can protect against noise induced stress.

Its deficiency (primary unlikely) occurs in patients with prolonged diarrhoea or vomiting and in patients on prolonged intravenous feeding. Its deficiency can lead to tetany, diabetes & heart problems (Includes hypertension, heart attack , ischemic heart disease).

(vii) Iodine

Sea foods are rich in iodine content. The recommended daily intake is 100mcg. perday in adults, which should be increased in children and pregnant & lactating women.

It is an essential component of thyroxine the hormone of the thyroid gland. In deficiency of iodine, the thyroid gland develops a swelling known as a "goitre". It is advisable to use iodised salt to increase the intake of iodine.

(viii) Copper

The rich source of copper is oystershel fish, rice and milk as well as use of copper utensels for cooking.

It is useful in myelin formation, melanin pigment synthesis, cholesterol metabolism, cardiac function, connective tissue synthesis, skeletal mineralization, immune factor and erythropoesis. Its deficiency can lead to microcytic hypercromic anaemia, depigmentation of hair & skin, skeletal demineralization and hypotonea.

(ix) Zinc

It is present in a wide variety of foods, but the main sources in diet are meat, milk, cheese, bread and cereals. The recommended intake is 15 to 30 mg. perday. The higher doses of zine may suppress immunity. Zinc functions as an antioxidant, and acts beneficially in wound healing. It is involved in large number of enzyme systems in the body and is essential for normal growth & development. Zinc also prevents toxic effects of cadmium, a heavy metal that pollutes the air, water & food. Zinc improves fertility. It also improves sperm count & sperm motility and protects prostrate gland against infection.

Its deficiency leads to stunted growth, loss of sence of taste, delayed sexual maturity, night blindness and in pregnancy can prolong labour.

(x) Cobalt

Traces of cobalt are present in many foods and its primary deficiency is unlikely in man.

Cobalt is a component of Vitamin B_{12}. It is, therefore, an essential dietary component which plays a role in blood formation.

(xi) Selenium

This mineral is vital for robust immunity. It acts as an antioxidant. It can suppress viruses, block cancer formation and protect the heart. The daily recommended intake is 50 to 200 mcg. perday. But excess intake can be toxic.

(xii) Chromium

We normally take traces of chromium in our diet but that is insufficient now a day's. The daily intake recommended is 200 mcg. per day. Probably in a 'biological active' form such as chromium picolinate.

Chromium plays vital role in regulating blood sugar. One of the great danger of age is excessive levels of blood glucose and blood insulin, which can bring on diabetes and other ills and generally destroy our health and shorten the life. Chromium normalises these factrors, lowers cholesterol and helps in preventing heart attack too.

Metabolism

It is a sum total of all biochemical processes which go on in the body and are essential for maintenance of normal life. Metabolism consists of two basic processes :-

Catabolism- The break down of complex molecules into simple products to liberate energy.

Anabolism- It is the synthesis of complex molecules from simple ones. Anabolic reactions require energy.

Thus the energy derived from catabolic reactions is used in anabolic reactions for the synthesis of complex molecules, muscular contractions, maintenance of body temperature, etc., as illustrated below:-

(i) Performance of mechanical work;

(ii) Maintenance of body temperature (98.6^{0}F or 37^0 C)

(iii) Functional activity of all glands, cells & tissues;

(iv) Synthesis of chemical substances, for the maintenance & growth of tissues and repair when required.

The break down of carbohydrates, proteins and fats in food occur in three stages. The first stage involves intestinal digestion and absorption of carbohydrates, proteins & fats. In the second stage, these substances are further broken down to give CO_2, H_2O, nitrogenous waste, three acids- acetic acid, oxaloacetic acid & alpha-ketoglutaric acid and some energy is liberated. And in the third stage, the three acids are oxidised completely (Kreb's cycle or citric acid cycle) and release a large amount of energy. The energy released is measured in calories. The energy liberated by catabolic processes in the body per unit of time is known as the "metabolic rate". Carbohydrates and protiens provides about 4 calories per gram & fats provides about 9 calories per gram.

A number of factors those affect metabolic rate, are sex, age, body size, climate, daily activity, muscular exertion, etc. The basal metobolic rate (BMR-measured under conditions of normal room temperature, physical & mental rest.) of an average sized man is 2000 calories per day. The daily diet for an adult requiring app. 2400 calories per day.

(a) Metabolism of Carbohydrates

The carbohydrates undergo digestion in the gastro-inestinal tract and are absorbed as monosaccharides - glucose, galactose & fructose. The galactose and fructose are converted into glucose in the liver and through the blood stream, glucose reaches in all the cells. Glucose is a major source of energy and used in the body in three ways:

(i) Broken down and oxidised to release energy

(ii) Stored as glycogen (In liver & skeletal muscles)

(iii) Converted in to fats and stored as fat.

In the presence of O_2, glucose/glycogen is broken down to pyruvic acid along with liberation of small amount of energy. Pyruvic acid is a metabolic stage reached by glucose or glycogen (carbohydrates), glycerol (fats) and many amino acids (proteins). In the presence of enzyme systems formed from thiamine (Vit. B_1), pantothenic acid & nicotinic acid, the pyruvic acid is converted into acetyl coenzyme -A. Acetyl coenzyme - A is further oxidised to release carbondioxide (CO_2), water (H_2O) and energy. The energy is stored in a compound called adenosine tri-phosphate (ATP) in the body.

Glucose can also be rebuilt from pyruvic acid & is stored in liver & skeletel muscles as glycogen. The process of formation of glycogen from glucose is called "Glycogenesis" and breakdown of glycogen to glucose is called "Glycogenolysis".

In case the glucose is present in the blood in excessive amount even after oxidation, is converted to fatty acids via pyruvic acid & acetyl coenzyme- A and deposited as fat (fatty acid + glycerol) in the body. The conversion of glucose to fat is promoted by insulin - a hormone secreted by the beta cells of the islets of langerhans (Pancreas). Where as glucose can be formed by glycerol liberated from digestion of fats and from amino acids after the amino group is removed known as - "Gluconeogenesis". The blood sugar level is kept within normal range in the body by Insulin (Pancreatic) as it lowers down when glucose level is high and by Hydrocortisone (Adrenal coretx), Adrenaline (adrenal medulla), Gulcagon (Alpha ceils of Pancreas), Thyroxine (Thyroid) & Growth hormone (Anterior Pituitary) as they increase glucose level in low serum glucose conditions.

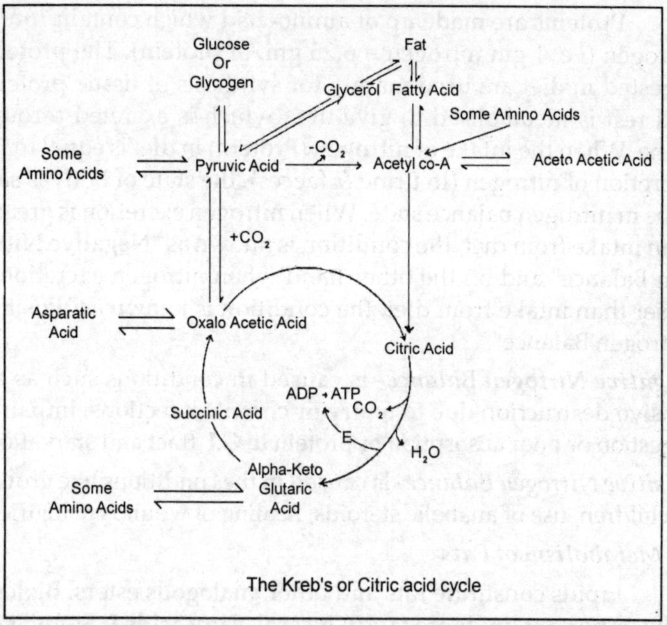

Fig.15

(b) Metabolism of Proteins

During digestion all proteins are broken down to amino acid and being absorbed from the intestine. The amino acids reach liver & other tissues via blood stream and are used in the body for synthesis of plasma proteins, proteins of various tissue cells, hormones, enzymes, antibodies etc. and utilized for the production of energy or converted to fat and / or carbohydrates in kreb's cycle. For the production of energy (kreb's cycle), the amino acids are deaminated in the liver as the amino group is removed by an oxidative process, which is converted to urea excreted in the urine and the remainder of the orginal amino-acid is available for oxidation and liberation of energy.

The cells of various tissues which are worn out due to age are continuously being replaced by newly formed cells. Only a small portion of amino acid of worn cells is lost from the body where as a large portion of amino-acid of worn cells (alongwith dietary amino-acid) is being reutilized for protein synthesis required for new cell & tissue formation.

Proteins are made up of amino-acid which contain 16% of nitrogen (i.e. 1 gm nitrogen = 6.25 gm. of protein). The proteins ingested in diet are used mainly for synthesis of tissue proteins and rest is metabolised to give urea which is excreted through urine. When the intake of nitrogen (Protein) in diet is equal to the excretion of nitrogen (In urine & faeces), the state of body is said to be in nitrogen balance state. When nitrogen excretion is greater than intake from diet, the condition is known as "Negative Nitrogen Balance" and on the other hand when nitrogen excretion is lesser than intake from diet, the condition is known as "Positive Nitrogen Balance".

Negative Nirtogen Balance- Is caused in conditions such as extensive destruction due to injury or chronic infections, impaired digestion or poor absorption of protein in G.I. tract and starvation.

Positive Nitrogen Balance- Is caused in the conditions like growth in children, use of anabolic steroids, healing of wounds & injuries.

(c) Metabolism of Fats

Lipids constitute fats and other analogous esters. Biologically important lipids are fats (Glycerol, Fatty acids & Stored fat). Fats are broken down in liver to glycerol and fatty acids. Glycerol is utilized by conversion into pyruvic acid. Fatty acids are oxidised to Acetyl co-enzyme-A, and enter the kreb's or citric acid cycle to release energy, CO_2 & water. The Acetyl co-enzyme-A may give rise to Acetoacetic acid in the liver, which along with beta-hydroxybutyric acid & acetone, forms a group of metabolically related substances known as "Ketone Bodies or Acetone Bodies". Any change which reduces the rate of carbohydrates oxidation in the liver will reduce the rate of complete oxidation of Acetyl coenzyme-A, without reducing the rate of its formation. Acetyl coenzyme-A is highly reactive and forms acetoacetic acid. The increase in the amount of acetoacetic acid which circulates in the blood leading to a condition known as "Ketosis". Ketosis can occur in starvation, diabetes and in people on a high fat low carbohydrate diet.

Cholesterol

It is a steroid widely distributed throughout the body. The main sources are (in diet) - egg, cream, butter, meat, liver, kidney & brain. It is not found in vegetable foods. The dietary cholesterol is absorbed from the intestines & deposited in the liver. It is also synthesized in the body mainly in liver from Acetylcoenzyme-A. It has been found that plasma cholesterol levels tend to be high on diet rich in saturatted fatty acids. A correlation has been found between high blood cholesterol levels and atherosclerosis (the hardening of the arteries) including coronary artery disease.

Nutritional Requirement & Deficiencies

The amount of nutrients sufficient for the physiological needs of an average healthy person is called the "Recommended Daily Allowance" (R.D.A.)

The nutritional deficiency is the state when a nutrient (vitamin or mineral) is not available in the body in adequate amount necessary for normal physiological functions. The nutritional deficiencies have been classified as (i) Primary deficiency that develops due to inadequate intake of nutrients in diet [causes are - poverty, war/famine, loss of appetite, in complete or wrong diet, consumption of polished rice, etc.], & (ii) Secondary deficiency - that develops due to inadequate availability of the nutrients in the body inspite of adequate amount being present in diet. [causes are physiological condition of a person, infections, fever, trauma, G.I. disorders, drug induced deficiencies and imbalance among nutrients, etc.]

Diet and Diseases

In diseases caused by deficiency of one or more nutrient factors, the obvious corrective measure is administration of deficient nutrients. Where as in the condition like impaired kidney function - may require restriction of proteins in diet; in the mangement of hypertension restriction of sodium in diet is beneficial and in diabetic subject restriction of carbohydrates in diet is necessary. So in the management of disease condition an appropriate diet is needed.

Clinical Aspects

Anabolic- Chemical substance which causes a synthesis of body protein.

Anaemia- A deficiency of haemoglobin concentration in the blood due to lack of R.B.C. and/or their haemoglobin contents.

Anti - Oxidants- The substances which protect against oxidative changes and damage caused by free radicals.

Beri-Beri- It is a deficiency disease caused by lack of Vit. - B_1. The common symptoms are muscular wasting, pain from (Neuritis), paralysis, progressive oedema, mental deterioration and at last heart failure.

Conjunctivitis- Inflammation of the conjunctiva.

Convulsions- Involuntary contractions of muscles due to many causes.

Diabetes- A disease characterized by polyuria. It is a conditon with hyperglycaemia due to diminished effectiveness or deficiency of Insulin.

Glossitis- Inflammation of the tongue.

Gout- It is a form of metabolic disorder in which sodium biurate is diposited in the cartilages of the joints (big toe), the ears and elsewhere.

Haemolysis- It is disintegration of red blood cells [R.B.C.] with liberation of haemoglobin.

Night Blindness (Nyctalopia)- It is a maladaptation of vision in darkness, may occurs in Vit. A deficiency.

Osteomalacia- It is infectious mineralization of the mature skeleton, with softening & bone pain. Commonly due to Vitamin - D deficiency.

Pellagra- A deficiency disease caused by lack of Vitamin - B complex (spl. Niacin) and protein.

Rickets- A disorder of calcium & phosphorus metabolism associated with a deficiency of Vit.- D, its beginning most often in infants & early childhood (between 6 month to 2 years).

Scurvy- A Vit. - C deficient disease characterised by pinpoint haemorrhage, oozing at the gums & fatigue.

Stomatitis- Inflammation of mouth (buccal mucous membrane).

Tetany- A condition of hyperexcitability where mild stimuli produces cramps and spasm.

Xerropthalmia- Dryness and ulceration of the cornea which may lead to blindness. It is associated with Vitamin -A deficiency.

Applied Medicines

(1) Tonics and Appetisers- Their main function is to stimulate appetite and they contributes to a feeling of well being.

Cyproheptadine-

Ciplactin (Cipla), Practin (Merind), Peritol (Themis Chem), Apetamin (Tablets India),Cydine (CFLPh.), Cyp-L (Albert David), Cypon (Geno)

Misc. Tonics- Bayer's Tonic (Bayer), Ferradol (Parke Davis), Hemiphos (Wyeth), Incremin (Wyeth), J.P. Tone (Jagson Pal), Kinetone Plus (Knoll), Nervitone (Alembic), Phosfomin (Sarabhai), Santevini (Novartis).

(2) Minerals and Nutritional Supplements-

Calcium-

Calcinol (Reptakos), Effcal (Eli Lilly), Shelcal (Elder), Richcal (Twilight), Trical - D (Sigma), Factocal (Wander), Magnical (Ethnor), Sovical (Solus) Cal. Sandoz (Novartis), Jactavit (Duphar), Ostocalcium (Glaxo), Calcindon (Indon), Dicalciplex (Khandelwal), Kalzana (German R.) Ossopan, Ossafez (TTK), Osex (Comed), Supracal (Pharmed)

Zinc-

Ulseel (TDPL), Zevit (SB), Zenbex-T (Abbott), Cobadex -Z (Glaxo) Vimez (Pharmacia), Becozinc (American R.), Zincovit (Apex).

Potassium-

Potklor (Walter B.), Potrelease (Natco), Potasol (Indoco), K-Gard (Wockhardt)

Amino Acids-

Aminodrip (Wockhardt), Hermin (Alembic), Vamin-G (Pharmacia)

Oral Electrolytes-

Electral (FDC), Electrobion (Merck), Emlyte (MM Labs), Peditral (R.P.G.), Relyte (Rallis), Ricetral (FDC)

Multivitamins-Minerals Combinations-

Multivite FM (Allenburys), Nutrisan (Novartis), Cyltabs (Duphar), Sharkoferrol (Alembic), Supradyn (Piramal H.C.), Beca Dexamin (Glaxo), Maxamin Forte (Anglo Fr.), Filibon (Wyeth).

(3) Vitamins-

Vit.-A-

Aquasol A (USV), Adexolin (Glaxo), Rovigon (Piramal H.C.)

Vit.-C-

Cecon Drops (Abbott), Celin (Glaxo), Chewcee (Cynamid), Redoxon (Piramal H.C.), Sorvicin (East India), Sukcee (IDPL).

Vit.-D-

Alpha D3 (Glaxo), Calcirol (Cadila), Rocaltrol (Piramal H.C.), Arachitol (Duphar)

Vit.-E-

Etoplex (USV), Evion (Merck), Evit (Abbott), Tocofer (Torrent)

Vit.-K-

K-Three Inj. (Medinex).

Vit.-B_1-

Benalgis (Franco Indian), Berin (Glaxo)

Vit.-B_2-

Lipabol (Cadila)

Vit.-B_6-

B-long (Elder), Pyricontin (Modi Mundi)

Vit.-B_{12}-

Macrabin (Glaxo)

Vit.-B_1, B_6, B_{12}:-

Bethadoxin-12 (B.E.), Neurobion (Merck), Sioneuron (Albert David)

Vit.-B Complex-

B.G.Prot (Merind), Becosules (Pfizer), Betonin (Knoll), Cobadex Forte (Glaxo), Eldervit (Elder), M.V.I.(USV), Optineuron (Lupin), Becozym-C (Piramal), Polybion (Merck), Sclerobion (Merck), Stresscaps (Wyeth), Vidaylin (Abbott),Visyneral (USV), Vitcofol (FDC), ABDEC Drops (Parke Davis), Basiton Forte (Sarabhai), Becadex (Glaxo).

Misc.-

Sporlac (Uni- Sankyo), Lactodex (Raptakos), Nutrolin -B (Cipla), Lactisyn (Franco Indian), Recupex (Wockhardt).

(4) Iron preparations- These are used as supplements in the treatment of iron-deficiency anaemia & as prophylactic in pregnancy, menorrhagia, infants, surgery and in malabsorption states.

Haemoglobin Preparations-

Dexorange (Franco Indian), Hepatoglobine (Raptakos), Haem-Up (Cadila Ph.), Hemfer (Alkem), Globac (Alidac).

Iron Formulations-

Fefol (S.B.), Autrin (Wyeth), Hepasules (B.E.), Iberol (Abbott), Tonoferon (East India), Livogan (Allenburys), Raricap (Ethnor), Dumasules (Pfizer), Softeron (Aristo), Vitcofol (FDC), Richfer (Twilight), Cheri (Indchemie), Orofer (Emcure)

Injectable Iron-

Imferon (Rallis), Jectofer (CFL Ph.), Neo-Hepatex (B.E.)

(5) Anabolics- They are the derivatives of testosterone and its main function is to help in cellular synthesis of proteins. Anabolic favours the increased retention of nitrogen, calcium, sodium, potassium, chloride and phosphates, leading to weight gain, water retention and increased growth of bone.

Oxymetholone-

Adroyd (Parke-Davis)

Stanozolol-

Menabol (CFL Ph.)

Nandrolone-

Durabolin and Deca-Durabolin (Infar), Metabol and Metadec (Jagson Pal), Neurabol and Deca Neurabol (Cadila H.C.), Protabol and Protadec(Macmillon), Neurophen and Deca Neurophen (Ind Swift).

(6) Anti-Obesity- (Appetite suppressants)

Fenfluramine-

Slimerax (Glaxo), Flabolin (Wockhart)

Dexfenfluramine-

Isomeride (Serdia)

(7) Food Products-

Protinex (Pfizer), Protinules (Alembic), GRD (Cadila H.C.), Promolan (Sarabhai), Trophox (Raptakos), Alprovit (Alkem), Prosan (Novartis), Soyal (FDC)

(8) Anti-Oxidants- They protects body against oxidative changes & damage caused by free radicals. Salace (Universal), Antoxid (American Rem.), Revup (Aristo),Orasca (Twilight), Ridase (Unichem), Oxigard (Glenmark), Oxyace (Unique), Revox

(Wallace), Socrit (Solus), Carnitor (Elder), Carnix (Twilight)

(9) Gout- Conditions of Hyper Uricaemia, a metabolic disorder.

Probenecid-

Bencid (Geno)

Allopurinol-

Zyloric (Wellcome),

Colchicine-

Goutnil (Inga), Kebutacine - I (Kee Pharma).

(10) Poisoning and Metabolic Dysfuction-

BAL Inj. (Knoll), Desferal (Novartis), Calcium Leucovorin (Wyeth), Glutaneurol (Franco-Indian), Lipigem (Torrent), Lipizyl (Nicholas), Lopid (Parke Davis), Rovacor (Stancare).

(11) Anti - Cancer-

Cholrambucil-

Leukeran (Wellcome)

Mustine Hcl-

Estracyt, Sterecyt (Merck), Mustine Hcl (Knoll).

Cisplatin-

Aquaplate (Khandelwal), Cisplatin (Biochem), Cytoplatin (Cipla)

Melphalin-

Alkeran (Wellcome)

Busulphan-

Myleran (Wellcome), Busuphan (Elder).

Lomustine-

Lomustine (Glaxo)

Mercaptopurine-

Mesna (German Rem.), Puri-Nethol (Wellcome)

Doxorubicin-

Adrim (Dabur), Doxorubicin (Khandelwal), Oncodria (TDPL)

Etoposide-

Bioposide (Biochem), Etosid (Cipla), Fytosid (Dabur)

Tamoxifen-

Nolvadex (ICI), Tamofen (Torrent)

Flutamide-

Drogenil (Fulford), Plutamide (Torrent)

Bleomycin-

Bleocin (Khandelwal), Bleomycin (Biochem), Oncobleo (TDPL)

(12) Immuno Suppressants- They are used to prevent transplant rejection and in the treatment of certain auto-immune diseases.
Azoran (R.P.G.), Imuran (Wellcome), Transimune (Troikaa)

Section- B

CHAPTER- 6

Blood, Lymph And Body Fluids

Blood

Blood is a connective tissue compound consisting of the blood cells or "Corpuscles" and plasma. In all 45% of the blood is occupied by blood cells and remaining 55% is plasma. Total volume of blood in an adult is about 5 litres. This blood volume remains relatively constant.

The Blood Cells- Three types of blood cells are found:

(1) R.B.C's. (Red Blood Cells or Erythrocytes),

(2) W.B.C's. (White Blood Cells or Leucocytes),

(3) Platelets (Thrombocytes).

(1) Red Blood Cells- The R.B.C's are circular, biconcave discs having about 7 microns in diameter. They contain haemoglobin in them. The matured R.B.C's have no nucleus. The total count per cubic millimetre of blood is about 5 million erythrocytes (4.5 to 5.5 millions cu. mm of blood). R.B.C's are formed in red bone marrow of flat and long bones with the help of protein, iron,Vit. B_{12} & folic acid and their lifespan is about 120 days.

The main function of R.B.C's is transport of gases with the help of haemoglobin. The normal amount of haemoglobin is 13.5 to 15.5 gram per millilitres of blood. Erthropoetin (produced by kidneys), Vit. B_{12}, Vit.-C, Folic acid & elements like Copper, Cobalt, Iron are necessary for R.B.C. production, (Erythropoiesis).

(2) White Blood Cells- They are white, larger & fewer in number than R.B.C's. The total count is about 6000 to 10000 W.B.C's per cubic millimetre of blood in normal adults. The W.B.C's are of two main types Granulocytes and Agranulocytes.

(a) Granulocytes:- They have many lobes & their protoplasm is granular. Available in 70 to 75% of the total W.B.C. count. Granulocytes are also known as Polymorphonuclear Cells. There are three types of Granulocytes

(i) Neutrophils (Phagocytes):- They are about 10 to 12 microns in diameter and these cells have a nucleus consisting 3 to 5 lobes with fine granular protoplasm. They form 60 to 70% of total W.B.C. count. Neutrophils engulf foreign particles, bacteria, dead tissues present in the blood & protect the body from invading micro-organism and help in elimination of foreign particles & dead tissue. The process of ingestion & digestion (engulf) by neutrophils is known as "Phagocytosis".

(ii) Eosinophils:- They are about 10 to 12 microns in diameter with a nucleus usually have two lobes. They are few in numbers and contributes 1 to 4% of total W.B.C. count.In worm infection & allergic conditions there number increases. Their function is not known.

(iii) Basophils- They have kidney shaped nucleus and found in few numbers. They contributes 0.5 to 2% of total W.B.C. count. Their function is not known.

(b) Agranulocytes- They contain no granules and are formed in the spleen & lymphatic tissue. There are two type of Agranulocytes

(i) Lymphocytes- They have large nucleus and cells are measuring 6 to 8 microns in diameter. They contribute about 20 to 30 % of total W.B.C. count. They do not possess phagocytic action but form antibodies. Lymphocytes are also believed to store, transport & release protein for the use by newly formed cells.

(ii) Monocytes- These are largest ones having about 15 to 20 microns in diameter with a kidney shaped nucleus. They contribute 4 to 8% of total W.B.C. count. They like neutrophils possess phagocytic action.

Leucocyte count- In different disease condition the total leucocyte count per cubic millimetre of blood is an important diagnostic aid. The % of each type of W.B.C. in the total count is known as the " Differential Count".

(3) Platelets- They are small cells, about 1/3rd of R.B.C. size with various shapes (oval, rod or spherical). The total count per cubic millimetre of blood is 2,00,000 to 4,00,000 Platelets.

Platelets are relatively fragile & break when subjected to any unusual mechanical stress. They contain an enzyme called 'Thrombokinase' which initiates clotting or co-agulation of blood. That's why they are also known as 'Thrombocytes'.

The Plasma- It is the intracellular fluid medium of blood consisting almost 91% of water, 7-8% of proteins, 0.9% salts and very small amount of glucose, fats, urea, uric acid, amino acids, the blood gases (O_2, CO_2 & N_2,), hormones & enzymes, etc. The pH of plasma is slightly alkaline and is constantly being maintained within a narrow range.

The plasma protein are of four main types Albumin, Globulin, Prothrombin & Fibrinogen. These proteins perform important functions. The albumin along with globulin helps in maintaining the colloid osmotic pressure of blood & thus helps in the maintenance of blood volume, & transport of material from blood to tissues and vice-versa. The globulin is composed of three fraction- alpha α, beta β, and gamma γ and contains antibodies of the body (specially gamma globulin). The prothrombin and fibrinogen plays vital role in the blood clotting.

Coagulation of Blood

(i) Extravascular clotting- During an injury when blood comes out of blood vessels, Thrombokinase is released from injured or broken platelets. Thrombokinase along with ionised calcium (which is present in blood), converts Prothrombin to Thrombin (active form). This active Thrombin further converts Fibrinogen to active Fibrin, which along with accumulated (dead blood cells) exudate forms a Fibrin barrier or Clot. The clot impaired microcirculation at injury site and resulted in inflammatory oedema. When the clot shrinks a straw coloured liquid or serum is squeezed out.

In the absence of ionised calcium, clotting can not occur, that's why when ever blood is collected and stored for transfusion or certain laboratory investigations - oxalate or citrate is added which in outsided blood vessels blood, forms non ionisable calcium, and thus blood can be prevented from clotting.

(ii) Intravascular clotting- Normally blood does not clot within blood vessels. During injury to blood vessel wall or/and slowing of blood flow in capillaries may lead to clotting of blood in the blood vessels. The clot inside the blood vessels is called as

"Thrombus" and the process of its forming is known as "Thrombosis".

Blood Groups- There are four groups of blood - A, B, O, and AB as illustrated below

Blood Group	Antigen in RBC	Antibodies in plasma
O	Nil	Anti-A + Anti-B
A	A	Anti-B
B	B	Anti-A
AB	A+B	Nil

Table - 2

The Rh factor is an antigen present in RBC's of about 85% population called 'Rh-positive' and absent in R.B.C.'s of rest population called 'Rh-negative'. Under normal circumstances, the Rh antibody (anti-Rh) is absent from the plasma of both Rh positive & Rh negative subject; but however can be formed in the plasma of Rh-negative individuals under certain conditions (in pregnancy) and may lead to a condition known as "Erythroblastosis foetails" (destruction of R.B.C.'s of the foetus).

Blood Transfusion

During or after severe blood loss or when erythrocyte count and haemoglobin count need to restore quickly, the bood is administred. The blood group A and group B can recieve blood from donors of their respective group and as well as of group-O; Group-AB (Universal receptors) as have no antibodies can recieve blood from any group; where as group-O which is universal donor can recieve blood from group 'O' only. The group's of reciepient and donor are tested by mixing the serum of the recipient with the R.B.C's of the donor by the process called "cross matching".

Lymph

The lymphatic system serves as one of the routes for removal of tissue fluid. It is also called as drainage system. The tissue fluid is the fluid present in the intracellular spaces. It is composed of the material passes out from capillaries of arteries and passing out to tissue cells. A large portion of tissue fluid flows back in to capillaries of veins and the remaining tissue fluid which is not removed enters a system of channels known as lymphatic vessels and is being now called "lymph".

The lymph is consisting of remaining tissue fluid, monocytes and lymphocytes. The lymph is carried by lymphatic vessels through lymph nodes back to the circulatory system. The lymph is milky in appearance as it contain fat absorbed from diet. The lymphatic vessels are thin-walled tubes extensively distributed through out the body and its tissues are made up of reticular tissue which contain precursors of lymphocytes. Lymphoid tissues may be dense (found in lymph nodes, tonsils, spleen) or diffuse (found in mucous membrane lining of G.I. tract & respiratory tract).

Lymph nodes are masses of lymphoid tissues, through which lymphatic vessels passes. Lymph nodes act as filters. Lymphatic system plays an important role in removing large substances such as proteins, bacteria, foreign particles, etc., which donot pass back into blood capillaries. At lymph nodes foreign particles & bacteria's are being engulfed by monocytes, thus preventing it from proceeding further. Lymph nodes also form lymphocytes, and antibodies and this function of lymph nodes are common to all lymphoid tissues.

Body Fluid

The body fluid consists of water of the body and its dissolved solutes. It is distributed in to two parts :-

(i) Intra Cellular Fluid (within the cells, app. 30 litres in an adult).

(ii) Extra Cellular Fluid (outside the cells, app. 12 litres in an adult).

The extra cellular fluid is made up of intracellular fluid, plasma of blood, digestive juices, urine, C.S.F., fluid of pleura and peritoneum, etc.

The intracellular or interstitial fluid is the medium in which the cells live, obtain food, O_2 & pass out the waste products through blood plasma. The body fluid can & does move from one compartment to the other. Normally the amount of fluid taken (through mouth) in to the body is same as the amount excreted (through lungs, skin, kidneys and only a small amount is lost in faeces). Under adverse conditions such as loss through vomiting, diarrhoea etc. and/or inadequate intake, the body makes adjustments to maintain plasma volume through other compartments. Kidneys through urine excrete fluid in variable amounts and establish a balance of intake and output to maintain 'fluid balance' of the body.

The electrolyte content varies between intracellular and extracellular fluid. Sodium is the main extracellular cation, Potassium is the main intracellular cation and Chloride is the chief anion of interstitial fluid. In the conditions like vomiting, diarrhoea, etc., loss of body fluid accompanied by loss of electrolytes can lead to disruption of acid-base balance. To restore normalcy the water and electrolyte replacement is neccessary up to the requirements, but not to over load the body with electrolytes.

Acid-Base Balance

The pH of blood and extracellular fluid is slightly alkaline (7.35 to 7.45) for the maintenance of large number of body functions. "Buffer system" which consists of weak acid (Carbonic acid) and its salts (Bicarbonate) helps to maintain the pH of blood and extracellular fluid. Disturbance of acid-base balance can lead to acidosis or alkalosis.

Acidosis is the condition when body gets an acid load, which can occur due to renal failure (renal acidosis), accumulation of ketoacids (diabetic acidosis), diarrhoea and depressed respiratory function (respiratory acidosis). In acidosis, the acid reacts with bicarbonate of the buffer system and forms carbonic acid, which is handled by - lungs, and is broken down to release water and CO_2, as well as by - kidney tubular cells to form ammonia, which helps to excrete H+ ions from carbonic acid and restore bicarbonate ions in the buffer system.

Alkalosis is the condition when body gets an alkali load. It can occur after excessive vomiting, ingestion of alkali for the treatment of peptic ulcer or urinary infections, in anxiety, fever,etc. In alkalosis the carbonic acid of the buffer system helps the formation of a weaker base.The lungs help to restore the balance by increasing in carbonic acid concentration and the kidneys by excreting large amount of bicarbonate.

A precise record of intake and output of fluids is important in a number of disease conditions such as-disorders of the kidney, congestive heart failure and in unconscious patients.

Clinical Aspects

Agranulocytosis- Complete absence or marked reduction in granulocytes or polymorphonuclear leucocytes.

Anaemia- A deficiency of haemoglobin concentration in the blood due to lack of R.B.C's and/or their haemoglobin contents. It is not a disease but a symptom of the underlying conditions. Causes of Anaemia:

(i) Due to diminished R.B.C. production

(ii) Due to blood destruction

(iii) Due to uncertain origins

(i) Due to diminished R.B.C. production

(a) Microlytic Hypochromic Anaemia:- Its main cause is iron deficiency.

(b) Megaloblastic or Pernicious Anaemia:- Its main cause is dificiency of VitaminB_{12} and folic acid resulting reduced number of R.B.C's count.

(c) Aplastic (Pancytopenia) Anaemia:- A condition where number of R.B.C, W.B.C. and Platelets are reduced due to aplasia of the bone marrow. It is of two types Primary Aplastic Anaemia (cause is not known) and Secondary Aplastic Anaemia (causes are radiation therapy, drugs like Amidopyrin, Chloramphenicol, etc., renal failure, chronic infections and chronic blood loss). Treatment is use of anabolics.

(ii) Due to blood destruction (Haemolytic Anaemia)

It is due to blood destruction, main causes are infection, malaria, leukaemia, drugs like Sulphonamides, Methyldopa, etc, elements like lead, radium, arsenic and hereditary abnormalities of R.B.C's.

(iii) Due to uncertain origins

Its causes may be chronic arthritis, renal failure, malignant disease, and chronic infections, etc.

Granulocytopenia- Decrease in number of polymorph or granulocytes.

Haematemesis- The blood vomiting.

Haematocele- A swelling filled with blood(Heamatoma).

Haematuria- Blood in the urine.

Haemoglobin- It is a respiratory pigment of R.B.C., composed of Haem(iron) and Globin (protein).

Haemophilia- Prolonged bleeding following even due to small injury, caused by deficiency of antihaemophilic globulin. It is an inherited disease found only in males.

Haemopoiesis- Formation of blood.

Haemoptysis- Blood in the cough.

Haemostatic- The agent which arrest or stop bleeding.

Leucocytolysis- Disintegration or distruction of leucocytes.

Leucocytosis- Increase in total leucocyte count. (e.g. in infections).

Leucopenia- Decrease in total leucocyte count.

Leukaemia- It is a malignant proliferation of the leucopoietic tissues with increase in leucocytes in the blood.

Lymphadenitis- Inflammation of a Lymph nodes.

Lymphangioma- A simple tumour of Lymph vessles.

Lymphangitis- Inflammation of a Lymph vessel.

Melaena- Black, tar-like stools. Evidence of Intestinal bleeding.

Applied Medicines

(i) Haem-a-Tonics-

Dexorange (Franco Indian), Haem-Up (Cadila Ph.), Heptaglobine (Raptakos), HB Plus (Torrent), Autrin (Wyeth), Fefol(SB), Hepasules (B.E.), Imferon(Rallis), Tonoferon (East India), Raricap (Ethnor), Iberol(Abbott), Hemsi (Serum), Jectofer inj (CFL), Softeron (Aristo), Richfer (Twilight), Cheri (Indchemie) , Orofer (Emcure), Eprex (Ethnor), Hemax (H.A.L.) Zyrop (Indon)

(ii) Anabolics-

Durabolin & Decadurabolin (Infar), Metabol & Metadec (Jagson Pal), Neurabol & Decaneurabol (Cadila HC), Protabol & Protadec (Macmillon), Neurophen and Decaneurophen (Ind Swift).

(iii) Haemostatics- These are the drugs which arrest or stop the bleeding.

Adrenochrome Monosemicarbazone-

Sigmachrome (Sigma), Siochrome (Albert David), Cadisper - C (Cadila), Kerutin - C (Mercury), Haemochrome (ACE), Stryptocid (Stadmed).

Aprotinin-

Aprogen (Bergen), Trasylolinf (Bayer)

Botropase-

Botropase (Juggat Ph.)

Ethamsylate-

Revici - E (Kee Ph.), Ethasyl (FDC), Dicynene (Dr. Reddy), Hemsyl (Indoco), Thams (Twilight), H-Stat (Obsurge), K-Stat (Mercury)

Diosmin & Bioflavonoid-

CVP & Gyne CVP (USV), Capimin (Helios), Daflon (Serdia), Venex (Elder), Venusmin (Martin & H)

Carboprost-

Prostodin (Astra - IDL)

Conjugated Oestrogens-

Premarin (Wyeth)

(iv) I.V. Fluids and Plasma Expanders -

Human Albumin-

Alubudec (Alidac), Albusafe (Win- Medicare)

Dextrose (2.5% to 50%), Normal Saline, 5% DNS, Ringer Lactate Sol.-

Available from - Albert David, Core, Krishna Keshav, PDPL, Mount Mettur.

20% Mannitol-

Core, PDPL, Unichem, Krishna Keshav, Albert David

Dextran-

Lomodex (Rallis), Plasmex (Core)

Polygeline-

Haemaccel (Hoechst), Seraccel (Serum).

Invert Sugar-

Fructodex (Raptakos), Fructocore (Core).

Electrolyte G/P/E/M/R-

Leclyte G/P/E/M/R (Albert David), PD-Lyte G/P/E/M (PDPL) Electrolyte G/P/E/M (Mount Mettur).

(v) Others- Cytarabine (Biochem),Cytocristin (Cipla), Oncotron (TDPL), etc, are available for leukaemia treatment (for more detail see chapter 5 of this section).

Section- B

CHAPTER- 7

Cardio-Vascular System

The cardiovascular system or circulatory system is the transport system of the body. It carries O_2 , nutrients & other substances to the tissues and excreted metabolic waste products. It is made up of:

(1) Blood (2) Heart (3) Blood Vessels

(1) Blood- The blood is a connective tissue compound consisting of the blood cells. The detail about blood has been described fully in chapter 6 of this section.

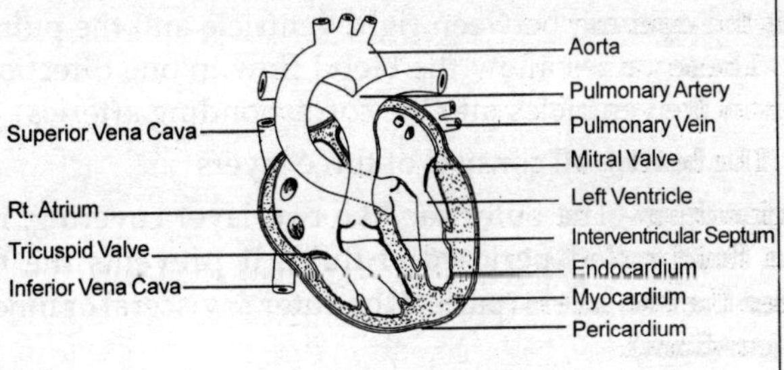

Structure Of Heart

Fig. 16

(2) Heart- It is a muscular pump which propels the blood. It is a hollow, muscular, cone-shaped organ lying in the chest between the two lungs. It is situated obliquely behind the sternum & adjoining parts of the rib cartilage. Two third of the heart is lying to the left of the midline. The heart pounds against the chest wall with each heart beat, which can be felt by the hand & is called the "Apex Beat". The size of heart is 12 cm. from base to apex, 8 to 9 cm. across and 6 cm. antero-posteriorly. It weighs about 300 grams.

The heart is divided into left and right halves by a muscular partition called "Septum". Each half is subdivided into two chambers - Artrium, the upper thin walled chamber and Ventricle, the lower thick walled chamber. Thus the heart contains the right artrium, right ventricle, left artrium & left ventricle.

Each artrium is connected below with the corresponding ventricle through an opening known as "atrio-ventricular orifice", which is guarded by valves known as "atrio- ventricular valves". The right valve has three leaflets or cups and is, therfore, known as "Tricuspid Valve" and the left valve has two leaflets or cups and thus is known as "Mitral Valve". Small, fine, fibrous cords proceed from the free edges of both the valves called "Chordae Tendinae" & attached to the papillar muscles, on the inner side of the ventricles. The function of artrio-ventricular valves is to allow blood to flow from the artrium to the ventricles but not in the reverse direction.

Two other valves are situated, one is at the base of aorta that leaves the heart from left ventricle and is known as "Aortic semilunar valve" & guards the opening between left ventricle & aorta, second one is at the base of pulmonary artery from right ventricle and is known as "Pulmonary semilunar valve" and guards the opening between right ventricle and the pulmonary artery. These valves allow the blood flow in one direction only, viz - from the ventricles into the corresponding arteries.

The heart wall consists of three layers

(i) Pericardium- The outer sac like two layer covering, is filled with a fluid called pericardial fluid. It prevents the friction between the two layers (parietal or outer & visceral or inner layer of pericardium).

(ii) Myocardium- The middle layer of the heart muscles consists of a special type of muscles known as "Cardiac muscles". The myocardium varies in thickness, it is thickest in the left ventricle & thinner in right ventricle. The myocardium has capacity to generate impulses spontaneously, which are responsible for the heart's rhythmic contractions and relaxations.

(iii) Endocardium- The inner smooth lining which lines the heart & is continued with the endothelial lining of the arteries & veins is composed of flat endothelial cells.

Heart Beat- The heart beats spontaneously and regularly about 70 times a minute in the resting adult. These properties of automaticity & rhythmicity are called intrinsic properties of the heart and are due to the modified heart muscle tissue, known as " intrinsic conducting system" which is capable of generating & conducting impulses within the heart. The intrinsic conducting system is comprised of the S-A node (sino-atrial node), A-V node (atrio-ventricular node) and Bundle of His & its branches.

The S-A node is situated in the upper part of the right atrium, A-V node is situated in the lower part of the right atrium & from it emerges the Bundle of His (atrioventricular bundle) which passes into the inter-ventricular septum and divides into two branches the right & the left branch. At last each branch divides in to fine fibres known as "Purkinje Fibres". The impulse normally initiates heart beat, arises in the S-A node (pace maker) and spreads through the atria & brings about atrial contraction. When the impulse reaches the A-V node, it spreads through the Bundle of His & Purkinje fibres to the ventricles and brings about ventricular contraction. Before the next impulse comes, the atria and the ventricles relax and get ready to contract again. The atrial contractions are weaker & of shorter period than the ventricular contractions.

Blood & Nerve Supply to Heart- The heart receives blood supply through the right and the left coronary arteries. They give rise to a net work of capillaries in the heart wall, and join to form coronary veins. These coronary veins unite and form the coronary sinus which drains into the right atrium.

The heart is supplied with autonomic nerves which regulate the rate & force of the heart beat (though not initiating it). There are two sets of nerves--

(i) Vagus nerves- Release acetylcholine and their stimulation, slow down the heart rate.

(ii) Sympathetic nerves- Release noradrenaline and their stimulation β receptor) & increase the rate and force of the heart beat. Both these nerves maintain a balanced heart rate.

(3) Blood Vessels

The blood vessels are hollow elastic tubes which carry blood to and from the tissue cells. They are of three types:

(a) Arteries- These are thick walled tubes and carry O_2 rich blood from the heart to various organs & tissues, with the exception of the pulmonary artery that carries impure blood to the lungs.

The aorta is the main artery, arises from the left ventricle, arches over the heart and passes behind it along the spine down through the thorax and the abdomen. It gives off branches to all the parts of body. The artery main branch divides into smaller branches, arteriols (the finest branch) and then end by joining the capillaries.

(b) Veins- These are thin-walled tubes and carry impure (oxygen poor) blood back to the heart from the organs & tissues, with the exception of the pulmonary veins which carry pure blood (O_2 rich) from the lungs to the left atrium of heart. The capillaries unite to form small veins known as venules, which unite further with other viens and form two principal veins- the "Superior Vena Cava", draining the head and neck and the "Inferior Vena Cava", draining the rest of the body, into right atrium of the heart.The veins have valves along their course which allow blood to flow towards the heart only.

(c) Capillaries- These are fine, microscopic vessels consisting of a single layer of endothelial cells & connect arteriols (artery) to venules (veins). The capillaries pass through nutrients, food, O_2 and water from blood to tissues and collect (reabsorbe) CO_2, water & waste products from tissues to blood.

Arteries & veins recieve post ganglionic sympathetic nerve fibres, which are adrenergic and release noradrenaline, when these nerve fibres are activated they stimulate alpha receptors in the muscle cells of the wall of blood vessels, leading to vasoconstriction (narrowing of blood vessels).

Cardiac Cycle & Cardiac Output

These are the events taking place in heart during one beat. The contraction of the heart or its chambers is known as "Systole" and the relexation is known as "Diastole".

The volume of blood pumped out by left ventricle in one minute is known as "Cardiac output". The cardiac output is app. 5 litres. There is increase in the cardiac output during exercise and emotional excitement. The cardiac output depends upon the volume of circulating blood, the efficiency of heart as pump and adequate return of blood to the heart from capillaries & veins.

Circulation of Blood

The circulation of blood from the heart to the various organs & back is generally of four types:

(i) Systemic Circulation- It comprises of the aorta & its branches, the capillaries and the veins. The circulation is made throughout the body organs practically.

(ii) Coronary Circulation- It is the part of systemic circulation but nourishes the heart itself. It differs from the systemic circulation as unlike other systemic artery, the coronary arteries fill up during diastole. The coronary arteries are of two types the right & the left, those further gives rise to a net work of capillaries in the heart wall and join to form coronary veins, which join to form coronary sinus, which drains into the right atrium. Any narrowing or blockage of a coronary artery has very serious consequences.

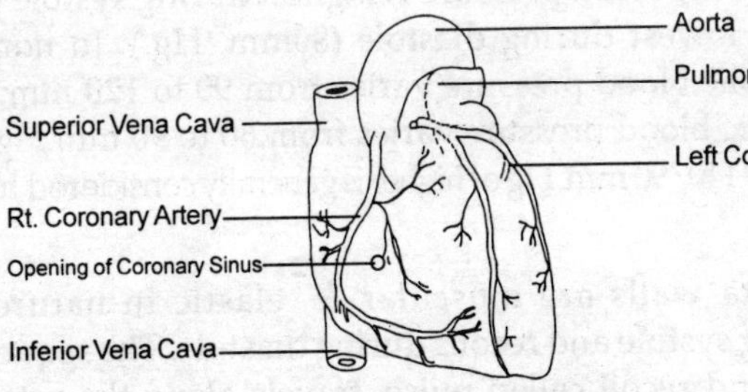

Coronary Circulation

Fig. 17

(iii) Pulmonary Circulation- It comprises of pulmonary artery & its branches (to carry impure blood from heart to lungs), the capillaries and the pulmonary veins (to carry pure blood from lungs to heart). The lung tissues recieve blood supply from systemic circulation only.

(iv) Portal Circulation- The veins which carry blood from the G.I. tract unite to form a large vein called the "Portal Vein", which enters the liver. The hepatic artery supplies the O_2 rich blood to liver. Both the portal vein & the hepatic artery divide in to a common network of capillaries and unite eventually to form the hepatic vein. The hepatic vein joins the inferior vena cava. The portal vein carries food materials, drugs absorbed from the G.I. tract to the liver, the hepatic artery mainly supplies O_2 for the metabolism of liver cells.

Blood Pressure

It is the force exerted by the blood on the walls of blood vessels and being generated by the pumping action of the heart. However, apart from the force of heart beat, it also depends on the volume of the blood present for circulation, the viscosity of blood, and the resistance offered by arteriols to the flow of blood.

The blood pressure is measured in millimetre of mercury (mm.Hg) by an instrument known as Syphygmomanometer. The blood pressure falls when heart beats feebly, the low blood volume due to injury, dilation of arteriols & dilation of capillaries & veins. The blood pressure increases during physical exercise, muscular work & emotional excitement.

The systemic blood pressure is highest during systole (120 mm. Hg.) and lowest during diastole (80mm. Hg.). In normal adult, the systolic blood pressure varies from 90 to 120 mm. Hg and the diastolic blood pressure varies from 60 to 90 mm.Hg . A blood pressure of 140/90 mm. Hg or higher is generally considered high.

The Pulse

The aorta walls are muscular & elastic in nature. It distends during systole and recoils during diastole. The sequence of distension and recoil called pulse, travels along the arteries and can be felt at several sites in the body, close to the surface and on artery lies over a bony prominence (commonly checked at the lower end of the radius bone). By feeling the pulse, a doctor can gain information about the heart rate, force of heart beat & a rough idea of the blood pressure. In a healthy adult the pulse rate varies from 60 to 80 per minutes (average 70 per minutes) during rest condition.

Clinical Aspects

Angina- Feeling of suffocation due to less O_2 supply to tissues.

Angina Pectoris- Severe but temporary attack of cardiac pain, which may radiate to the arms, caused due to defficient blood supply to myocardium.

Angioma- A non-malignant tumour formed in blood vessels.

Aortic Regurgitation- Incompetence of the valve with back flow.

Atherosclerosis- A degenerative arterial change associated with advance age and co-exist with deposition of hard yellow lipoid material in the intimal layer of the arteries.

Bradycardia- Slow rate of heart contraction resulting slow pulse rate.

Cardiac Arrhythmias- Disease involving the specialized conducting system of the heart gives rise to various abnormalities of rhythm; known as cardiac arrhythmias or dysrhythmias.

Congestive Heart Failure- The unability to pump out all the blood, receives from the veins, by diseased heart muscle; the condition is known as CHF (Cardiac Heart Failure)

Coronary Thrombosis- Complete blockage of a narrowed coronary artery by a clot.

Dyspnoea- Difficulty in breathing.

Endocarditis- Inflammation of the endocardium.

Hypertension- Rise of blood pressure generally above 140/90 mm. Hg.

(i) Primary Hypertension- The condition when no definite cause is found for the rise of blood pressure. It is also known as "Essential Hypertension".

(ii) Secondary Hypertension- The condition when cause is known for the rise of blood pressure.

Hypotension- Excessive fall in blood pressure generally below 90/60 mm. Hg.

Ischaemia- Lack of adequate blood supply to tissues.

Ischaemic Heart Disease(IHD)- Narrowing of one or more coronary arteries. It is also known as coronary heart disease (CHD).

Mitral stenosis- Narrowing of the mitral orifice, usually due to rheumatic fever.

Myocardial Infarction- Death of a section of cardiac tissue due to lack of blood supply.

Oedema- Abnormal infilteration of tissues with fluid.

Palpitation- Rapid forceful beating of the heart, the patient is concious.

Pericardial Effusion- Accumulation of fluid in the pericardial cavity.

Pericarditis- Inflammation of the pericardium.

Tachycardia- Excessive increase in heart rate.

Applied Medicines

A large number of medicines are availabe for the management of cardio-vascular disorders, viz.- Anti hypertensive, Antianginal, Antiplatelets, Anti thrombotics and Anticoagulant, etc. Few of them (brand names) are written below

(1) Thiazides- They initially induce a sodium and water loss leading to a fall in plasma volume & extracellular fluid, which in trun lowers the cardiac out put & blood pressure

Hydrochlorothiazide & Benzthiazide-

Esidrex (Novartis), Biduret (Glaxo), Ditide (S.B.)

Chlorthalidone-

Hythalton, Clothalton (S.P.P.L.)

(2) Beta-Blockers- The β1 receptor produces cardiac stimulation, where as β2 receptor produces bronchodilation & vasodilation. Nonslective betablockers antagonise all the beta adrengic effect, whereas slective betablockers antagonise the β1 cardiostimulatory effects.

Nonslective Beta-Blockers

Propranolol-

Betabloc (USV), Ciplar (Cipla), Inderal (ICI), Tensyn (Synokem)

Pindolol-

Visken (Novartis)

Sotalol-

Sotagard (Glaxo)

Oxprenolol-

Trasicor (Novartis)

Carvedilol-

Cardivas (Sun), Carvil (Zydus), Caslot (Stancare)

Slective Beta- Blockers

Metoprolol-

Betaloc (Astra IDL), Metolar (Cipla), Selopres (Astra-IDL)

Atenolol-

Atelol (Themis Pharma), Betacard (Torrent), Tenolol(IPCA), Tenormin (ICI), Atecard (Dabur), Atecard-D (Dabur), Dibeta

(Torrent), Atelol -D (Themis Pharma),Tenoclor (ICI), Tenoric (IPCA), Angitol (Ind-Swift), Atenova (Lupin)

Acebutolol-

Sectral (Rhone-Poulenc)

Bisoprolol-

Concor (Merck), Corbis (Unisearch)

Celiprolol-

Celicard (USV), Celipres (Solus)

Esmolol-

Miniblock (USV)

Labetalol-

L-Beta (Plethico), Normadate (Glaxo)

(3) ACE Inhibitors- They inhibit the angiotensin converting enzyme (Kinase II) involved in the conversion of angiotensin I to angiotensin II. They also cause direct arteriolar vasodilation.

Captopril-

Aceten & Acezide (Wockhardt), Angiopril (Torrent), Captopril (Lupin)

Lisinopril-

Cipril (Cipla), Lisoril (IPCA), Zestril (ICI)

Enalapril-

BQL (Cadila H.C.), Envas (Cadila Pharma), Minipril (Alembic), Enace & Enace-D (Nicholas), Vasopril (Protec)

Ramipril-

Cardace (Hoechst), Ramace (Astra IDL)

Perindopril-

Coversyl (Serdia)

Losartan-

Alsartan (Aristo), Losar (Unichem), Repace (Sun)

(4) Calcium Channel Blockers- They reduces the magnitude of the calcium current in the sino-atrial (S-A) & atrioventricular (A-V) nodes by blocking the slow inward calcium channels. Also used to treat angina.

Verapamil-

Isoptin (German Remedies), Vasopten (Torrent)

Nifedipine-

Calcigard (Torrent), Depin (Cadila H.C.), Myogard (R.P.G.), Nicardia (Unique), Beta-Nicardia (Unique), Angiblock (Alkem), Betanif (Unichem), Presolar (Cipla), Tenofed (IPCA)

Diltiazem-

Angizem (Sun), Dilcardia (Unique), Dilzem (Torrent), Diltisyn (Themis Ph.) Dilgard (Protec), Cardem (A.F.D.)

Felodipine-

Felogard (Cipla), Renedil (Hoechst)

Nitrendipine-

Cardif (Concept), Cardif Beta (Concept), Nitrepin (USV)

Benidipine-

Caritec (Stancare)

Amlodipine-

Tamlod (Merind), Topdip (R.P.G.), Amcard (Systopic), Amlopres & Amlopres- AT (Cipla), Stamlo & Stamlo Beta (D.R.L.), Amlovas (Macleods), Amlosafe (Genetica)

(5) Nitrates- They reduces preload & after load and can be used as adjunctive therapy to diuretics & cardiac glycosides in the management of congestive heart failure. The vasodilation effect of nitrates produces headache & facial flushing which diminishes with time. They also relieve angina.

Isosorbide Dinitrate-

Isordil (Wyeth), Sorbitrate (Nicholas)

Isosorbide-5 Mononitrate-

Ismo (Knoll), Monit (Intas), Monotrate (Sun)

Glyceryl Trinitrate-

Angised (Wellcome), Nitrocontin (Modi Mundi), Nitroderm TTS (Novartis), Myovin (Cadila)

Erythrityl Tetranitrate-

Cardilate (Wellcome)

Pentaerythritol Tetranitrate-

Peritrate (Warner)

(6) Vasodilators- Normally they block alpha adrenergic receptors and produce vasodilation. Some increase blood flow of the microcirculation due to histamine like activity and some produce more dilation of the blush areas than the extermities.

Isoxsuprine-

Duvadilan (Duphar), Suprox (Ind-swift), Udilan (Troikaa), Tidilan (Juggat)

Xanthinol Nicotinate-

Complamina (German Remedies)

Pentoxifylline-

Flexital (Sun), Trental (Hoechst), Erytal (Recon)

Nylidrin Hcl-

Arlidin (USV)

Nicorandil-

Nikoran (Torrent), K-Cor (Macleods)

Cinnarizine-

Cintigo (Wallace), Stugeron (Ethnor)

(7) Antihypertensives- These drugs reduces high blood pressue.

Clonidine-

Arkamin & Arkamin-H (Unichem), Clothalton (S.P.P.L.), Catapres (G.Remedies)

Methyldopa-

Alphadopa (Merind), Emdopa (IDPL)

Reserpine-

Adelphane & Adelphane esidrex (Novartis)

Prazosin-

Minipress-XL (Pfizer), Prazopress (Sun)

Terazosin-

Hytrin (Abbott), Olyster (Cadila H.C.)

Indapamide-

Lorvas (Torrent), Natrilix (Serdia)

Lacidipine-

Lacivas (Sun), Sinopil (Glaxo)

(8) Drugs in cardiac failure & shocks

Digoxin-

Digoxin (Wellcome), Digox (Cadila), Lanoxin (Wellcome), Digitran (Macleods)

Mephentermine-

Mephentine (Wyeth)

Dopamine-

Dopamine (TTK), Dopinga (Inga)

Dobutamine-

Dobutrex (Eli Lilly), Dobucin (Troikaa), Kardia (Panacea)

(9) Antithrombotics- They increase the amount of the proteolytic enzyme plasmin by raising the circulating level of its precursor plasminogen.

Streptokinase-

Embokinase (Modi Mundi), Streptase (Hoechst)

Urokinase-

Urokinase (Modi Mundi & TTK), Ukidan (Serum)

Tissue Plasminogen Activatior-

Actilyse (German Remedies)

(10) Antiarryhythmics- These are used to control or cure cardiac arrhythmias, which are caused by disorders of electrical impulse generation and / or by disturbance in impulse conduction.

Quinidine-

Quinidine (Wellcome), Quininga (Inga)

Procainamide-

Pronestyl (Sarabhai)

Amiodarone-

Aldarone (Alidac), Panarone (Panacea)

Disopyramide-

Norpace (R.P.G.), Regubeat (Glaxo)

Lignocaine-

Gesicard (S.P.P.L.), Xylocard 2% (Astra IDL)

Amiodarone-

Aldarone (Alidac), Panarone (Panacea)

Mexiletine-

Mexitil (German Remedies)

Propafenone-

Rhythmonorm (German Remedies)

(11) Antiplatelets- They reduce platelet adhesion and aggregation and can be useful as prophylactic meaures to prevent clot formation.

Dipyridamol-

Dynacard (USV), Persantin (German Remedies), Cardiwell, Cardiwell plus (Torrent), Dynasprin (USV),

Aspirin-

ASA-50 (G-Remedies), Disprin and Colsprin-100 (R.C.I.), Asalite (Twilight), Aspent (Solus), Delisprin (Aristo)

Ticlopidine-

Ticlovas (U.S.V.) Tikleen (IPCA), Tyklid (Torrent)

(12) Anticoagulants- They antagonise the effects of vitamin -K by interfering with their synthesis in the liver.

Warfarin-

Uniwarfin (Unichem)

Heparin-

Beparin Inj. (B.E.), Declot (Recon), Lomorin (VHB)

Acenocoumarol-

Acitrom (S.P.P.L.)

Reviparin-

Clivarine (Knoll)

Enoxaparin-

Clexane (R.Poulenc)

Section- B

CHAPTER- 8

Respiratory System

The respiratory system serves us the function of breathing. It is divided in to:

(a) Upper Respiratory Tract- Consisting of the nasal cavity, the paranasal sinuses, the nasopharynx and the larynx.

(b) Lower Respiratory Tract- Consisting of the trachea, the bronchi, & bronchioles and the lungs.

(c) The Pleura, the muscles for respiration and the nerves & nerve centres which control respiration, can be considered as accessary, but essential components of the respiratory system.

Functions- The functions of the respiratory system are

(i) Inspiration - to take O_2 rich air in to the lungs,

(ii) Expiration - to expel out the CO_2 loaded air from the lungs.

The mechanical function of inspiration & expiration is known as ventilation; which is being influenced by the potency of the respiratory passages & the function of respiratory muscles. The exchange of O_2 and CO_2 between the inhaled air & blood flowing through lungs is called "External Respiration". And the exchange of gases between the blood & tissues is called "Internal Respiration". The act of breathing or respiration comprises ventilation and the external respiration.

(a) Upper Respiratory Tract

(i) Nasal cavity- The nasal cavity is situated between the skull cavity above and the oral cavity below and is divided length wise in two halves with a partition known as "Nasal Septum"; consisting of partly of bone & partly of cartilage. Each half of the nasal cavity opens in front to the exterior, and behind it opens into the nasopharynx. The external opening or nostrils are lined by skin covered cartilage (Alaenasi) which is rich in hair follicles, that act as filters to catch dust particles in the inhaled air. The upper parts of nasal cavity are lined by the olfactory epithelium and functions as the special sense organ.

The lateral walls of the nasal cavity have three bony ridges,the superior, the middle and the inferior conchae & are running from front towards the rear. Each conchae forms a roof over a tunnellike passage known as meatuses (a superior, a middle & an inferior), & running along the length of lateral wall. The sinuses (frontal & maxillary-open at middle meatus, sphenoidal & ethmoidal - open at superior meatus) open at meatus, the nasopharynx begins along with opening of eustachian tube at the rear end of the middle meatus. The nasal cavity as whole lined by a thick, carpet like ciliated epithelium & is richly supplied with blood vessels.

Functions- The mucus secretion of the nasal cavity help to increase the moisture content , the rich blood supply help to warm up the inhaled air and entangle the escaped dust particles & smoke from nostrils. Thus the air that enters the lungs is made moist, warm & free from foreign particles. The paranasal sinuses act as resonators of the nasal sound of speech.

(ii) Paranasal Sinuses- It contains two frontal sinuses, two maxillary sinuses, a sphenoidal sinus and a group of ethmoidal sinuses. The sinuses are lined with ciliated epithelium and open into the nasal cavity.

Functions- The mucous membrane of the sinuses provides a large surface area to facillitate the moistening & warming up of inhaled air. It also acts as resonators of the nasal sound.

(iii) Pharynx- It is situated behind the posterior openings of nasal cavity and continues below.The space behind the nasal cavity is called "Nasopharynx" and the space behind the oral cavity is called "Oropharynx". The lateral wall of Nasopharynx contain opening of the Eustachian tube and the posterior wall contains adenoid (a collection of lymphatic tissue). The oropharynx communicates below with the oesophagus and above with the larynx (Laryngopharynx). On either side of the oropharynx are situated two oval gland-like structures of lymphoid tissue known as the "Tonsils".

Functions- It act as a common communicating space between the nasal & oral cavity and the oesophagus & larynx. The adenoid and tonsils exerts protective function by rounding up any pathogenic micro organisms that attempt to invade either the digestive or the respiratory passages.

(iv) Larynx- It is also called as voice box, consists of a frame work of cartilage lined by ciliated epithelium. It connects with the laryngopharynx above, with the trachea below. The upper opening of larynx is called "Glottis", is guarded in front by a cartilagenous tongue like structure called "Epiglottis". The middle of larynx has two longitudinal folds of mucous membrane known as "Vocal Cords", which contain a strip of voluntary muscle inside.

Functions- The primary function of larynx is to act as an organ of speech; and a part of the air passage. Secondly to prevent the food from entering the larynx (& trachea) during swallowing of meal.

(b) Lower Respiratory Tract

(i) Trachea, Bronchi & Bronchioles- The trachea or "Wind Pipe" begin at the lower end of larynx and extends downwards at ends divided in to two branches called the "Bronchi" a right and a left for each lung. The each bronchus is divided in to smaller tubes, and the finest one is known as "Bronchioles". The walls of trachea are lined by ciliated epithelium & secrecte mucus continuously. The outer surface of the trachea consists entirely of smooth muscle; and in between it contains rings of cartilage, which are incomplete where the oesophagus is in close contact with the trachea. These rings of cartilage are joined together by intervening smooth muscle tissue.

The structure of the bronchi is similar to that of the trachea, except that the cartilaginous rings become smaller & smaller; where as the walls of bronchioles are devoid of cartilage and consist of smooth muscles only.

The trachea, the bronchi and the bronchioles constitute the "Tracheo-Bronchial Tree", which provides a passage for the air.

Functions- The mucus secreted by the walls of tracheo- bronchial tree moisten & warm the air, and is constantly propelled upwards alongwith the foreign and dust particles, towards the larynx by its ciliary movement; and induce the protective reflex action of cough.

(ii) Lungs- The lungs are two in number, a right and a left, situated in the thoracic cavity. The lungs are surrounded completely except the hilum, by the layer called pleura. The right lung is divided in to three lobes; upper, middle & lower. The left lung contains only two lobes; an upper and a lower. Each lobe of both the lungs is further divided into small functional units called "Broncho Pulmonary Segments".

In each segment the bronchioles divide into finest tubes which finally open into small air sacs or "Alveoli".

Each alveolus has a two layered wall, the outer layer, consisting of capillary endothelium and the inner layer, consisting of squamous, non-ciliated respiratory epithelium. The space between the alveoli contains loose connective tissue & elastic tissue which help lungs to expand during inspiration, and contract during expiration.

Functions- The main job of the lung is external respiration. O_2 from the inhaled air diffuses from the alveoli into the capillary blood and CO_2 from capillary blood into the alveoli and then expel out. Thus lungs which recieve O_2 poor blood from the right ventricle, send back O_2 rich blood to the left ventricle.

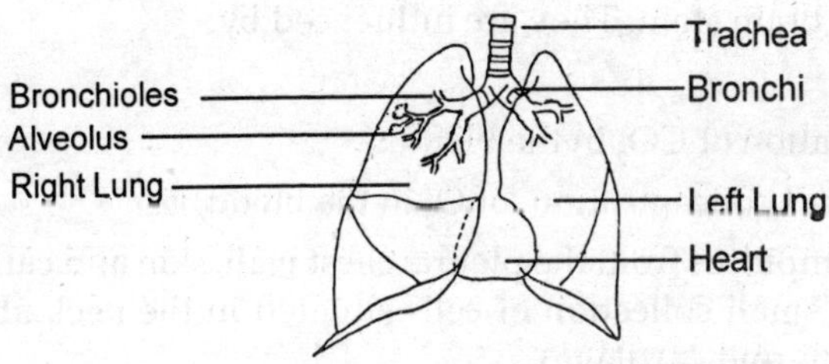

The Lower Respiratory Tract

Fig.18

(iii) Pleura- It is a two layered envelop that surrounds each lung completely except the region [where the main bronchi and the pulmonary blood vessels enter it] called the "Hilum". The outer layer of pleura that is in close contact with the chest wall is called "Parietal Layer" and the inner layer that is in close contact with the lung is called "Visceral layer". The pleural sac is filled with a fluid called "Pleural Fluid", that facilitates the movement of the visceral and the parietal layer against each other during expansion & contraction of the lungs.

The pleural sac provides a protective covering for the lungs and help lungs to expands during inspiration.

(iv) Muscles of Respiration- The muscles of respiration are

(a) The Diaphragm- It is a dome - shaped sheet of skeletel muscle separating the thoracic cavity from the abdominal cavity;

(b) The Intercostal muscles- They join the ribs together and form a part of the chest wall ;

(c) The Accessory muscles- It consist the muscles of the neck & chest & are attached to the chest wall.

The muscles of respiration help in the act of respiration by pulling the chest wall and rib cage outward to initiate inspiration and help the chest wall to contract passively during expiration.

(v) The Nerves- The diaphragm is supplied by two nerves, the phrenic nerve and the intercostal nerve; the intercostal muscles receive motor fibres through the intercostal nerve, and the accessory muscles are supplied by their respective spinal motor nerves.

The respiratory movements are controlled by a centre called "Respiratory Centre", which is located in the pons & medulla oblongata of brain stem. They are influenced by:-

(a) Emotions,

(b) Concentration of CO_2 in the blood,

(c) A decreased concentration of O_2 in the blood, &

(d) Sensory impulses from the pleura, chest wall, skin and cartoid body (It is a small collection of cells situated in the neck at the level of the thyroid cartilage).

Cough Reflex

Whenever a foreign particle tries to enter the lower respiratory tract, it is thrown out by a series of violent expiratory bouts called the "Cough". The cough is a reflex response induced not only by foreign irritants, but also by inflammation in the respiratory passage, accumulation of respiratory secretions & irritation of the pleura or pharynx.

Clinical Aspects

Acute Pulmonary Oedema- The acute left ventricular failure leads tocongestion and plasma then escapes into alveoli and interferes with proper respiration. Symptoms are - coughs, breathlessness & bloodtinged sputum.

Asthma- Paroxysmal airway's obstructon due to generalized narrowing of the bronchi.

Bronchial Asthma- Attack of breathlessness associated with bronchial obstruction or spasm.

Bronchiectasis- Dilatation of the bronchial tubes following repeated infections.

Bronchiolitis- Inflammation of the bronchioles.

Bronchitis - Inflammation of the bronchi, may be acute or chronic.

Cyanosis- Appearance of bluish colour, especially in the mucus membrane of the mouth, the conjuctiva and the nail beds.

Dyspnoea- Difficulty in breathing.

Hypoxia- Diminished amount of O_2 in the tissues.

Laryngitis- Inflammation of the larynx.

Mucoviscidosis- Failure of development of normal mucus secreting glands, sweat glands & pancreas. It is a congenital hereditary disease, common in infants with septic bronchitis & steatorrhoea.

Nasopharyngitis- Inflammation of the nasopharynx.

Nasosinusitis- Inflammation of the nose and adjacent sinuses.

Pleuritis (Pleurisy)- Inflammation of the pleura. It is of two types; viz - Dry pleurisy and pleurisy with effusion.

Pneumonia- Inflammation of the lungs, with production of alveolar exudate. It is of 4 types viz. - lobarpneumonia, Bronchopneumonia, Hypostaticpneumonia, & unresolved pneumonia. It is usually due to the infection by micro - organism.

Pulmonary Emphysema- A condition of alveolar distension accompained with chronic bronchitis or partial obstruction of a bronchus or bronchiole.

Respiratory Failure- The failure of the lungs to oxygenate the blood adequately.

Rhinitis- Inflammation of the nasal mucus membrane.

Sinusitis- Inflammation of a sinus (usually paranasal sinuses).

Sputum- The matter which is expectorated from the lungs.

Status Asthmaticus- Repeated attacks of asthma without any period of freedom between spasms.

Tonsillitis- Inflammation of the tonsils.

Tracheitis- Inflammation of the trachea.

Applied Medicines

(1) Antiasthmatics (Bronchodilators)- The parasympathetic system causes bronchoconstriction mediated by acetylcholine. The sympathetic stimulation mediated by noradrenaline causes increased pulmonary blood flow, bronchodilation and vasodilation of the pulmonary circulation. The humoral factors include histamine, serotonin, bradykinin, etc., cause broncho constriction.

(i) Sympathomimetic amines

(a) Drugs stimulating alpha & beta receptors

Adrenaline, Ephedrine.

(b) Drugs stimulating $beta_1$ & $beta_2$ receptors

Isoprenaline, Orciprenaline

(c) Drugs stimulating $beta_2$ receptors

Salbutamol, Terbutaline.

The beta adrenergic agonists cause bronchodilation by promoting the formation of C-ATP and this in turn relaxes the bronchial muscle.

Ephedrine-

Alergin (Cipla), Asmapax Depot (Nicholas), Asmotone (East India)

Isoprenaline-

Isoprin (Unichem), Neo-Epinine (Wellcome)

Orciprenaline-

Alupent (German Remedies)

Salbutamol-

Asthalin (Cipla), Bronko (Glaxo), Ventorlin (Glaxo), Brokosyrup (Glaxo), Grinlinctus-BM (Franco)

Terbutaline-

Bricanyl (Astra IDL), Asmotone plus (East India), Terpect (Themis Chem), Theobric (Astra IDL).

(ii) Xanthine derivatives- The xanthines producing smooth muscle relaxation including bronchodilation, by inhibiting

the enzyme phosphodiesterase.

Aminophylline-

Aminophylline (Wellcome), Cortasthma (Cadila H.C.), Sedonal (East India).

Theophylline-

Theo PA (Wellcome), Theolong (SOL), Unicontin (Modi mundi), Cadiphylate Elixer (Cadila H.C.), Deriphyllin(G-Remedies), Tedral (P. Davis), Theobid (Protec), Phylin-I (Obsurge), Broncordil (Neo Ph.)

(iii) Mast cell stabilisers- These drugs prevent the release of chemical mediators of bronchoconstriction from sensitised mast cells and reduce bronchial hyper reactivity.

Ketotifen-

Asthafen (Torrent), Tritofen (FDC), Zerosma (Merind)

Sodium Cromoglycate-

Cromal (Cipla), Fintal (Rallis), Ifiral (Unique).

(2) Antitussives- The antitussives depress the cough centre in the medulla of brain, resulting in an elevation of the cough threshold. In high dose may cause respiratory depression. Commonly used antitussives are Codeine, Ethylmorphine(narcotic antitussive), Dextromethorphan, Noscapine (non-narcotic antitussive), Chlophedianol (peripherally acting), etc.

Codeine-

Codeine sulphate, Dionindon, Codinlinctus (Indon), Glycodin terp vasaka (Alembic), Mit'slinctus (Astra-IDL), Phensedyl cough linctus (Rhone Poulenc).

Chlophedianol-

Detigon linctus (Bayer).

Dextromethorphen-

Actifed DM (Wellcome), Corex DX (Pfizer), Ephedrex (Alembic), Deletus (Nicholas), Zeet linctus (Alembic), Tuspress (Indoco), Tuxiril (Medley), Xecof (Morepen)

Noscapine-

Coscopin Linctus (B.E.), Tuxyne (Franco-Indian).

(3) Expectorant and mucolytic agents- These agents alter the viscosity of the sputum and promote the removal of secretions from the bronchial tree.

Expectorants-

Avil Exp. (Hoechst), Dilosyn Exp. (Allenburys), Phensedyl Exp. (Rhone Poulenc), Piriton Exp. (Glaxo), Toxoril (Twilight), Tuspel Plus (Indoco), Terpect Exp. (Themis Chem), Xpar, (BombayTab.), Norvent (Indcheme), Sudex (Comed)

Mucolytics-

Bisolvon (G. Remedies), Bromhexine (IPCA), Mucodyne (Elder), Bidanzen (Glaxo), Serato-M (Kee Pharma), Solvin (IPCA), Cheston (Protec), Seratid (Twilight)

(4) Cough mixtures- Benadryl cough formula (Parke Davis), Clistin (Ethnor), Coscopin plus, Coscopin-BR(B.E.), Grilinctus (Franco-Indian), Lupihist (Lupin), Viscodyne (Tata), Zedex (Wockhardt).

(5) Decongestants- Benadryl (Parke Davis), Sudafed (Wellcome), Corex (Pfizer), Tixylix cough linc. (Rhone Poulenc), Triaminic (Wander), Actifed plus (Wellcome), Cinaryl (Themis Pharma), Dristan (Wyeth), Febrex plus (Indoco), Rinostate (Searle), Pedia-3 (Ethnor), Zadine-maxi (Fulford), Sinarest (Centaur)

(6) Corticosteroids- Beclate Inhaler (Cipla), Betnelan (Glaxo), Wysolone (Wyeth), Walacort (Wallace), Dexona (Cadila H.C.), Decdan (Merind), Predicort (Macmillon), Deltacortil (Pfizer).

(7) Respiratory stimulants- Doxapram (Khandelwal) is a non -specific analeptic agent used to stimulate respiration. It is used rarely as temporary measures to correct acute respiratory insufficiency in chronic obstructive lung disease.

(8) Inhalers and nebulizers- Aerocort (Cipla), Asthalin (Cipla), Bricanyl (Astra IDL), Fintal (Rallis), Salmete R (D.R.L.), Salbutamol (Allenburys), Azrol (Natco), Brovon (Glaxo), Budecort (Protec).

Section- B

CHAPTER- 9

Genito - Urinary System

It comprises of the urinary system and the reproductive system.

(a) Urinary System

The urinary system is concerned with the formation and excretion of urine. The main organs are-two kidneys, two ureters, the urinary bladder and the urethra.

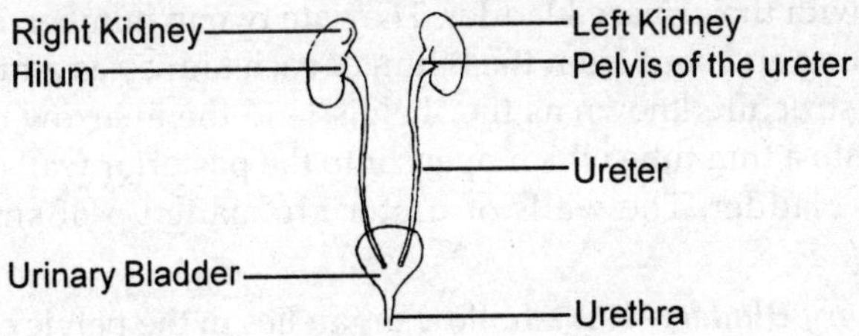

The Urinary System.

Fig.19

(1) Kidneys- They are two in number, having bean shape & measuring each about 10 cm. long, 5cm. broad and 2.5 cm. thick. They are situated on the either side of vertebral column, on the posterior wall of the abdominal cavity, behind the peritonium, and at the level of the last thoracic and the upper three lumbar vertebrae.

The kidney is made up of a large number of microscopic units called the "Nephrons". The kidney is divided into two zones, the outer one is called "Cortex" and the inner one is called "Medulla".

Each nephron consists of "Glomerulus", surrounded by a funnel-like structure called "Bowman's Capsule", which further extended to the "Renal tubule". The renal tubule is divided into the "Proximal convulated tubule", the u-shaped "Loop of Henle" and the "Distal convulated tubule", which finally joins a "Collecting tubule", that collects urine from a number of renal tubules.

On the middle border of each kidney is a slit like opening, the "Hilum",through which pass the blood vessels of the kidney and the ureter.

Each kidney receives blood supply through the renal artery, which enter in it through the hilum and divides into branches.

The smallest branch the "Afferent arteriole", enters a Bowman's Capsule and from the glomerulus (a tuft of capillaries), then it is taken away by the "Efferent arteriole",which divides into a second set of capillaries surrounding the renal tubule. The efferent capillaries lead to small veins, and finally unite to form the "Renal Vein".

(2) Ureters- The ureter is a tube like structure, connecting each kidney with the urinary bladder. They are two in number, about 25 cm. long and start from the hilum of each kidney as a funnel-shaped structure known as the "Pelvis" and then narrow down below into a thin tube which opens into the posterior wall of the urinary bladder. The walls of ureter are made up of smooth muscles.

(3) Urinary Bladder- It is a hollow organ lies in the pelvic cavity behind the pubis. The upper part of urinary bladder is known as "Fundus" and the lower end is fixed in position . In the male, it lies just in front of the rectum, & in the female it lies just in front of the uterus. The walls of the urinary bladder consist of mucus membrane (Inner lining), muscular (middle lining) and fibrous tissue (outermost lining). The urinary bladder opens downward into the urethra. The urinary bladder acts as a reservoir of urine. The usual capacity of the bladder is about 300-350 ml., but under certain circumstances the bladder can get distend to hold upto 800 ml. of urine.

(4) Urethra- It is a canal starting from the bladder to the external opening which is called as "External urinary meatus". Urethra is lined with mucus membrane.

The male urethra is about 20 cm. long and passes through the prostate gland, pelvis muscles, and the entire length of the penis. It act as a common passage for the urinary as well as the reproductive system.

In female the urethra is short, straight, about 5cm. long and lies just in front of the vagina. It serves as a passage for urine only. As female urethra is short and opens close to the anus, the chances of urinary tract infections are more in them compare to the males.

Urine- The urine is light yellow coloured clear solution formed in the kidneys. Depending upon the amount of fluid intake about 1 lit. to 1.5 lit. of urine is excreted in a day. The urine has slightly acidic pH (around 6); but varies in different infections/disease conditions.

Urine is composed of mainly water (96%), urea (2%) & sodium chloride. Besides a number of electrolyte derived from the diets, water soluble vitamins, enzymes, hormones and urochrome are also excreted in the urine, but in small amounts.

The kidneys form urine and help our body to get rid of liquid waste materials, depending upon the fluid intake and thus maintain water and electrolyte balance in our body. Basically three processes are involved in the formation of urine :-

(i) Filtration- The wall of glomerular capillaries & Bowman's capsule serve as a filter and the plasma containing all the salts, glucose & other small molecules are filtered through them.

(ii) Reabsorption- The filtered fluid passes through the three segments of the renal tubules, where the cells of the tubule reabsorb those substances that are required by the body viz-a large portion of water, sodiumions, chloride ions, glucose & uric acid, etc.,and leave behind those that are not required by the body.

(iii) Secretion- The tubular cells secrete some materials directly into the filtrate viz-secretion of H+and K+in exchange of Na+, ammonia, metabolic products-creatinine, glucuronic acid and number of foreign substances including drugs, etc.

Substances which are passed out into the urine fall into two groups:

(a) Threshold substances- e.g. glucose, normally not present in the urine.

(b) Nonthreshold substances- e.g. urea, creatinine, foreign substances are always present in the urine.

Micturition- It is the act of passing urine. The desire to pass urine is due to an increase in pressure inside the bladder caused by increasing accumulation of urine. It is a reflex action controlled by reflex arc present in the bladder wall. If the opportunity to void urine does not present itself, the bladder can hold a large quantity of urine. It is also controlled by higher centres situated in the cerebral cortex, basal ganglia & reticular formation.

Incontinence means passage of urine without any control, caused due to loss of control of higher centres, weakness of the sphincters, narrowing of urethra and in male due to prostatitis.

Functions of the Kidney

The main functions of the kidney are:

(a) Removal of waste products (viz-urea, drugs, toxins, etc.),

(b) Maintenance of water & electrolyte balance in the body,

(c) Regulation of the acid-base balance.

(B) Reproductive System

The purpose of the reproductive system is to bring forth springs and ensure continuation of the species. It can be divided in to

(1) Primary Sex Organs (Gonads)- Testes in male and ovaries in female.

(2) Secondary Sex Organs- These can be divided into the internal organs & the external organs.

Male Reproductive System

(1) Primary Sex Organs- Testes.

(2) Secondary Sex Organs-

(i) Internal - Epididymis, Vasdeferens, Seminal Vesicles and Prostate gland.

(ii) External- Penis and Scrotum.

Structure of Male Reproductive System

The testes are two in number and situated in the "Scrotum", which is a pouch of skin. Each testis is enclosed in a two layered sac of thin serous membrane, called "Tunica". Microscopically, the testes consist of a large number of fine tubules, called

"Seminiferous tubules", which produce the male reproductive cells or spermatozoa under the influence of FSH (Follicle Stimulating Hormone). These fine tubules join one another & form a large coiled tube, called "Epididymis", which continues as the "Vasdeferens". The "interstitial cells" (Leyding cells) are situated in between the seminiferous tubules and produce the male sex hormone, called "Testosterone" under the influence of ICSH (Interstitial Cell Stimulating Hormone) & pour it into the blood.

The Vasdeferens begins as a continuation of the epididymis, is thick, cord-like tube enters the pelvic cavity, runs behind the urinary bladder & join the other vasdeferens to form the ejaculatory duct.

The Seminal Vesicles are two oblong sac situated behind the bladder and open into ejaculatory duct via its ducts.

The Prostate gland is a small structure situated behind the bladder and contain a large number of tubular glands. The ducts of tubular glands open into the prostatic urethra.

The Urethra is about 20cm. long in male, which begins at the lower end of the bladder & passes through the Prostate gland, the Perineal muscles & the Penis.

The Penis is a tubular structure covered with skin. The body of Penis is composed of three cylindrical bands of spongy, vascular, erectile tissue, which are extended into the perineum and are attached to the pelvic bones. The Glans Penis is a bulb-like structure covered with a retractable fold of skin, called "Foreskin or Prepuce". The Urethra opens on the Glans Penis. The sexual arousal & erection of the Penis are under hormonal as well as neural & psychologic controls.

Functions

(i) Production of spermatozoa, which is essential for male fertility.

(ii) Production of Testosterone, which is responsible for the development & maintenance of secondary sexual characters (External genitalia, growth of moustache & beard, growth of pubic hair, breaking of the voice at puberty).

(iii) The Seminal Vesicles secrete a fluid which nourishes to the spermatozoa.

(iv) The Prostate glands secrete a fluid which also nourishing to the spermatozoa & adds to the volume of the seminal fluid.

(v) The Urethra acts as a common pathway for urine as well as semen.

Female Reproductive System

(1) Primary Sex Organs- Ovaries

(2) Secondary Sex Organs

(i) Internal- Fallopian tubes, the Uterus & the Vagina.

(ii) External- Vulva, Labia majora, Labia minora & the Clitoris.

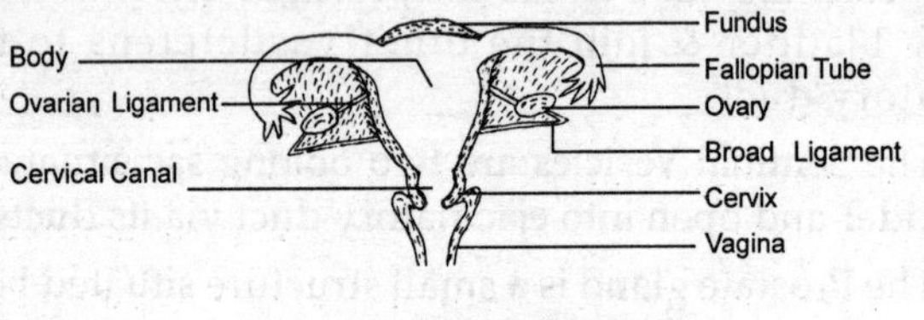

Female Internal genital organs

Fig. 20

Structure of Female Reproductive System

The Ovaries are two almond sized oval bodies situated on either side of uterus in the pelvic cavity. They are attached to the uterus by means of a fibrous cord called "Ovarian Ligament" and are enveloped in a double layer of the peritoneum known as the "Broad Ligament". Microscopically, the ovary is seen to contain a large number of spherical structures called "Primordial follicles". One of these follicles grows and matures into a "Graafian follicle" every month from puberty to menopause and contain the "Ovum" (female germ cell).

The Fallopian tubes are 10 cm. long muscular ducts extending from the ovaries to the uterus. They have finger-like structure called "Fimbrae" towards the ovarian ends, which facilitates the entry of the ovum into fallopian tubes by ciliary movement during ovulation. The fertilization of the ovum takes place in the ampulla region of the fallopian tube.

The Uterus is a pear-shaped organ situated in the midline of the pelvic cavity & between the bladder & the rectum. It can be divided into three parts, the upper one called as "Fundus", the middle portion is called as "Body"and the lower most portion is called as "Cervix", which communicate inside towards the body with "Interal Oss" and outside towards the vagina with "External Oss". The wall of uterus consist of thick muscular three layers viz. "Peritoneum", "Myometrium" and "Endometrium (lined with a sponge -like mucous membrane).

The Vagina is a fibro-muscular passage leading from the Cervix to the Labia minora. It is lined by stratified squamous epithelium which is richly supplied with blood vessels and mucous glands.

The Vulva consists of two thick folds of skin, the "Labia majora"and the "Labia minora". The Labia minora surround the vaginal opening (Introitus) and the "Clitoris", a small nodule of erectile tissue. The vaginal orifice is partially covered by a thin diaphragm/membrane known as"Hymen" (especially in young girls). Two large mucus-secreting glands called "Bartholin's glands", are situated on either side of the introitus.

The Urethra in females is much shorter than male and is about 5 cm. in length, and its opening is situated in front of the vaginal opening, behind the clitoris. The mass of tissue & skin situated between external genitals and anus is known as "Perineum". It stretches to a remarkable extent during labour.

Functions

(i) The ovaries produces ovum and secretes hormones-Oestrogen and Progestrone.

(ii) The uterus receive the fertilized ovum and retained it during pregnancy. It expel out foetus at the end of pregnancy by the contraction of its muscular wall in response to Oxytocin hormone. The uterus also plays part in the phenomena of mensturation.

(iii) The vaginal epithelium relatively resistant to bacterial and protozoal infections.

Ovulation:

The ovary contains many thousands of ova called "Primary-Oocytes" and are lie dormant until the onset of puberty. Each ova is surrounded by a cluster of follicles. At each menstrual cycle (about the 5th day of cycle), one follicle in the ovary begins to grow and mature under the influence of "Follicle Stimulating Hormone" (FSH) of the anterior pituitary, at the same time it secretes a hormone"Oestradiol", which stimulates the endometrium of uterus to grow and become thick. The follicle becomes fully matured in about 10-14 day's & becomes progressively larger and gradually migrates to the surface. Due to increasing pressure, the full grown graafian follicle ruptures and releases the ovum under the influence of the "Luteinising Hormone" (LH) of the anterior pituitary and the ovum is discharge into fallopian tube. This process of rupture of graafian follicle is called "Ovulation". The residual mass of graafian follicle after the expulsion of ovum is called "Corpus Luteum",which secretes the hormone "Progesterone" and brings about proliferation of glands in the endometrium (Secretory Phase).

Menstruation

The female reproductive system undergoes cyclic changes at intervals of about 28 days known as "Menstrual Cycle". It is, a phenomena where cyclic bleeding occurs after about 28 days because of periodic shedding of the progestational endometrium. The menstrual cycle start at 'Monarch'(onset of menstruation after puberty) and end at 'Menopause' (cessation of menstruation around 45 years of age). It is absent in pregnancy & lactation, or because of some endocrine disorder. First day of the bleeding is taken as first day of cycle. The first half of the mensturation (Day 1 to 14th) is under the influence of Oestrogen hormone and called "Proliferative stage", the second half of the cycle is mainly under the influence of Progesterone hormone as well as of Oestrogen and called "Secretory phase".

If fertilization of the ovum doesnot occur, the Corpus Luteum begins to shrink around the 24th day and the secretion of Oestradiol as well as Progesterone rapidly falls. Owing to lack of hormonal support , the thickened endometrium begins to disintegrate, break down and bleed. Thus the menstrual flow begins at the end of day 28 and a new cycle begins.

Fertilization

It is the impregnation of an ovum by a spermatozoon. The fertilization takes place in the fallopian tubes. After fertilization the fertilized ovum travels very slowly towards uterus & implanted in the uterus about 10 day's after the fertilization and begins to grow. The Progesterone makes endometrium suitable for implantation of the ovum. In this case the Corpus Luteum does-not shrink, but increase both in size and activity (continues to produce Oestradiol & Progesterone throughout the period of pregnancy). The fertilized ovum carries 23 pairs of chromosome of which one pair is sex chromosome either XX (Female) or XY (Male).

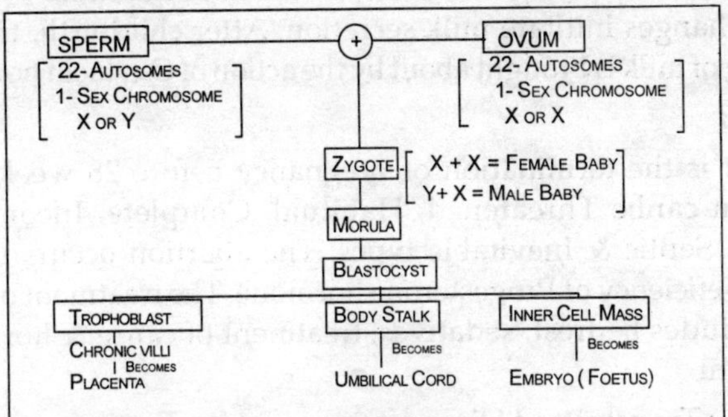

The Fertilization

Fig. 21

Pregnancy

If fertilization takes place, the ovum gets implanted into the endometrium and multiplies to form the embryo, from which the foetus eventually develops. As the foetus grow, so does the uterus. The average duration of pregnancy in humans is 280 days.

The placenta is an organ in which blood vessels of embryo & later of the foetus are brought in the intimate relationship with the blood of the mother. The placenta serves the function of Nutrition, Respiration, Excretion, Barrier to infections and secretes Hormones (viz.H.C.G., H.P.L., Oestrogen, Progesterone) & Enzymes (viz. Histaminase, Oxytocinase), which are very much important for the successful maintenance of pregnancy. The placenta takes over the production of hormones (Oestrogen & Progesterone) from the Corpus Luteum around 100th day of pregnancy.

Pregnancy makes the mother prone to anaemia, urinary tract infections & vaginal infections. Administration of drugs during pregnancy (especially during the first three months) requires the probable benefits to the mother be weighed against possible adverse effects on the foetus.

Mammary Glands

The mammary glands or breasts are regarded as secondary sex organs. They begin to develop at puberty under the influence of Oestradiol hormone. During pregnancy the continued production of L.H. and the Progesterone hormones, brings about secretory changes in the epithelium of mammary glands. These changes inititate milk secretion. After childbirth, the outpouring of milk is brought about by the action of Oxytocin hormone.

Abortion

It is the termination of pregnancy before 28 weeks. The abortion canbe Threatened, Habitual, Complete, Incomplete, Missed, Septic & Inevitable types. The abortion occurs mainly due to deficiency of Progesterone hormone. The treatment of abortion includes bedrest, sedatives, treatment of cause & hormonal treatment.

Sexually Transmitted Diseases

These includes followings:

(i) Syphilis- It is caused by the spirochaete "Treponema pallidum". Clinically, three stages of syphilis are recognised.

The primary lesion is a round painless ulcer on external genitals, called "Hard Chancre". Although the infection appears to be superficial, the T. pallidum spread rapidly through out the body via the lymphatics and if not treated may damage the cardiovascular and the nervous system after a few years.

(2) Gonorrhoea- It is caused by the gonococcus or "Neisseria gonorrhoeae".

In the male it gives rise to urethritis , prostatitis, and/or epididymo-orchitis.

In the female it gives rise to bartholinitis, vaginitis, cervicitis and salpingitis.

(3) Trichomoniasis- It is a protozoal infection caused by "Trichomonas vaginalis".

It causes vaginitis in the female and urethritis in the male.

(4) Chancroid- It is caused by a gram negative bacillus, "Haemophilus ducreyi".

It produces painful ulcers (Soft Chancre) on the genitalia.

(5) Non-gonococcal Urethritis- It may be caused by "Chlamydia trachomatis and Mycoplasma hominis".

(6) Genital Herpes-It is caused by "Herpes simplex virus", characterised by genital ulcers in women and blisters or ulcers in men.

(7) Lymphogranuloma Venereum- It is caused by the "Chlamydia", characterised by the enlargement of inguinal lymph nodes which may suppurate and break down to produce ulcerating lesions.

(8) Granuloma Inguinale- It is caused by a gram-negative organism "D. granulomatis", characterised by a proliferative lesion on the genitalia.

(9) Mollusa Contagiosa- It is an infectious type of wart which appears on the skin as a pearly papules, with an umbilicated centre of molluscum contagiosum on the lower abdomen and thighs.

Clinical Aspects

(A) Urinary system

Albuminuria- The presence of albumin in the urine.

Anuria- Absence of urine formation by the kidneys.

Catheterization- Insertion of catheter, usually into the urinary bladder.

Chronic renal failure- The continue falls in the glomerular filteration rate, below normal.

Cystitis- Inflammation of the urinary bladder, usually due to bacterial infections.

Globulinuria- The presence of globulin in the urine.

Glomerulonephritis- The non-suppurative inflammation of the glomeruli.

Haematuria- The presence of R.B.C. or blood in the urine.

Nephropyosis- The pus formation in the kidney.

Nephrosis- Any degenerative, non-inflammatory changes in the kidney.

Nephrotic Syndrome- The term used as synonym for type-II nephritis, leading to albuminuria, oedema & heavy proteinuria.

Nephritis- The inflammatory or an inflammatory-like reaction, diffuse, in the kidney.

Nocturia- Passing of the urine at night.

Pyelitis- The mild form of pyelonephritis with pus in the urine.

Pyelonephritis- The infection involving the kidney's cortex and pelvis.

Pyuria- The presence of pus in the urine.

Renal Calculas- The stone in the kidney.

Renal Oedema- The abnormal infiltration of tissue with fluid, as a result from disturbed kidney filtration in nephritis.

Renal Colic- The spasm of ureter due to a stone.

Uraemia- The retention of urea and other nitrogenous substances in the blood, due to kidney dysfunction of various causes.

Ureteritis- The inflammation of a ureter.

Urethritis- The inflammation of the urethra.

(B) Reproductive system

Abortion- It is the termination of pregnancy before 28 weeks.

Amenorrhoea- The absence of the menses.

Balanitis- Inflammation of the glans penis and perpuce (Balanoposthitis).

Bartholinitis- Inflammation of Bartholin's glands.

Castration- The removal of the testicles in the male or the ovaries in the female.

Cervicitis- Inflammation of the cervix.

Cryptorchism- It is a devlopmental defect, whereby the testes don't desend into the scrotum.

Dysmenorrhoea- The painful menstruation.

Endometriosis- Inflammation of the endometrium.

Failure of Nidation- The failure in implantation of the early embryo in the uterine mucosa.

Fertilization- The impregnation of an ovum by a spermatozoon.

Gynaecomastia- Enlargement of the male mammary gland.

Hydrocele- A swelling due to accumulation of the serous fluid in the tunica vaginalis of the testes, or in the spermatic cord.

Impotent- The absence of sexual power in male.

Infertility- The lack of ability to reproduce.

Labour- The act of giving birth to a child.

Lactation- The period during which the child is nourished from the breast.

Leucorrhoea- A sticky, whitish vaginal discharge.

Mastitis- Inflammation of the the breast.

Menopause- The cessation of menstruation, occuring normally between the ages of 45 and 50.

Menorrhagia- An excessive & prolonged menstruation.

Menstruation- The flow of blood from the uterus, occurs for 4 to 5 days after every 28 days in the female.

Metritis- Inflammation of the uterus.

Metorrhagia- The uterine bleeding between the menstrual periods.

Metropathia haemorrhagica- Irregular episodes of uterine bleeding due to excessive oestrin in the blood stream. Usually associated with a follicular cyst in the ovary.

Orchitis- Inflammation of the testicle.

P.I.D.- The inflammatory reaction in the pelvic organs & their surrounding connective tissues due to infections, called pelvic inflammatory disease.

Phimosis- Tightness of the prepuce so that it cannot be retracted over the glans penis.

Prostatitis- Inflammation of the prostate gland.

Salpingitis- Inflammation of the fallopian tubes.

Trichomoniasis- Inflammation of the vagina in females and of the urethra in males, caused by Trichomonas vaginalis.

Uterine Inertia- The lack of contraction of parturient uterus.

Vaginitis- Inflammation of the vagina.

Vulvitis- Inflammation of the vulva.

Vulvovaginitis- Inflammation of the vulva and vagina.

Applied Medicines

(1) Diuretics and Antidiuretics- The diuretics are the drugs which increases the flow of urine. Where as antidiuretics are the durgs which reduces the volume of urine.

Amiloride-

Amifru-40 (Elder), Frumil (Geno), Lasiride (Hoechst)

Triamterene-

Ditide (S.B.), Frusemene (S.B.)

Acetazolamide-

Diamox (Wyeth), Actamide (Micro)

Hydrochlorothiazide-

Esidrex (Novartis), Biduret (Glaxo)

Frusamide-

Lasix (Hoechst), Salinex (IDPL)

Spironolactone-

Aldactone, Aldactide, Spiromide (R.P.G.), Fruselac (Lupin), Lasilactone (Hoechst), Lactone (Sun)

Xipamide-

Xipamid (German Remedies)

(2) Alkalisers- They provide symptomatic relief during the U.T.I., by raising the pH of the urine and thereby counter acting the burning sensation of an acidic urine.

Disodium Hydrogen Citrate-

Citralka (Parke Davis), Cital (Indoco) Oricitral (TTK), Alkanil (Inga), Dicetral (Samson), Syntral (Synokem)

(3) Urinary Antiinfective/Antiseptic

Nitrofurantoin-

Furadantin (S.B.), Trifuran (MM Lab.).

Nalidixic Acid-

Gramoneg (Ranbaxy), Ulix- P (Blue Cross), Negadix (CFL Ph.)

Cotrimazine-

Aubril (Novartis), Silizine (B.E.) Triglobe (Astra IDL)

Cotrimoxazole-

Bactrim (Piramal H.C.), Oriprim (Cadila H.C.), Septran (Wellcome), Synastat (Roussel)

Methenamine-

Mandelamine (Parke Davis).

(4) Urinary Analgesics and Antispasmodics

Phenazopyridine-

Pyridium (Warner), Pyridactil (Ethnor)

Dicyclomine-

Meftal spas (Blue Cross), Spasmindon (Indon), Colimex (Wallace), Cyclopam (Indoco), Spasmo-Proxyvon (Wockhardt)

Flavoxate-

Urispas (Walter Bushnell), Flavoxate (Elder)

(5) Drugs Acting on Uterus-

Ergometrine-

Ergacap (Mercury), Ergotab (Jagson Pal)

Methylergometrine-

Satergin (Tablet India), Utergin (Sigma), Methylergometrine (Novartis), Ergolin (Lincoln)

Carboprost Tromethamine-

Prostodin (Astra IDL)

Dinoprostone-

Cerviprime, Primiprost (Astra IDL)

Ritodrine-

Yutopar (Duphar), Ritodine (Troikaa)

Ethacridine Lactate-

Emcredil (M M Lab.), Vecredil (Jagson Pal)

Isoxsuprine -

Duvadilan (Duphar), Suprox (Ind-Swift), Udilan (Troikaa)

Oxytocin-

Gynotocin (Sigma), Pitocin (Parke Davis), Syntocinon (Novartis)

(6) Fertility Agents, TropHic Hormones, Androgenic Steroids & Related Drugs-

Menotrophin-

Metrodin (Serum), Pregnorm (Win-Medicare)

Gonadotrophin-

Gonadotrophin L.H. (Biochem), Humegon (Infar)

Bromocriptine-

Parlodel (Novartis), Proctinal (Glaxo)

H.C.G.-

Corion (Win-Medicare), Gonotrop-C (Modi Mundi), Ovidac (Alidac), Choriomon (Panacea), Pregnyl (Infar)

Testosterone-

Testanon, Sustanon (Infar), Testoviron (G.Remedies), Aquaviron (Piramal H.C.)

Mesterolone-

Provironum (G.Remedies), Restore (B.B.)

Danazol-

Gonablok (Win-Medicare), Gynazol (Sun), Zendol (Serum)

Allyloestrenol-

Fetugard (Glaxo), Anin (Ind-Swift), Maintane (J.P.), Profar (Infar)

Conjugated Oestrogen-

Premarin (Wyeth)

Clomiphene-

Fertotab (Glaxo), Ovofar (Infar), Fertomid (Cipla)

Ethinyloestradiol-

Evalon, Mixogen (Infar), Progynon (G. Remedies), Estogen (Macmillon), Lynoral (Infar), Estraderm TTS (Ciba)

Ethyloestrenol-

Orabolin (Infar)

Medrooxyprogesterone-

Farlutal (Pharmacia), Primolut-N (G. Remedies)

Hydroxyprogesterone Caproate-

Proluton Depot (G. Remedies), Maintane Inj. (Jagson Pal), Anin Inj. (Ind-Swift)

Norethindrone-

Regesterone (Novartis), Styptin (G.Remedies)

Dehydroprogesterone-

Duphaston (Duphar)

(7) Contraceptives-

Oral-

Centron (Torrent), Saheli (Kerala Drugs), Duoluton-L (G.Remedies), Orgalutin (Infar), Ovral (Wyeth), Triquilar (G. Remedies), Novelon (Infar)

Spermicidal-

Delfen Cream (Ethnor), Ortho-Gynol Vag. Jelly (Ethnor)

(8) Drugs for Vaginal & Urethral Conditions-

Miconazole-

Gyno-Dektarin (Ethnor), Zole Ovules (Rexel)

Ciclopiroxolamine-

Batrafan Cream (Hoechst), Larpox Vag. (Lyka)

Clotrimazole-

Candid (Glenmark), Canesten Vaginal (Bayer), Gynostatum (Crossland), Imidil Vag. (Lyka), Gynotrim (Sigma)

Povidone Iodine-

Betadine Sol. & Passaries (Win-Medicare), Alphadin Sol. & Passaries (Nicholas), Wokadine Vag. (Wockhardt)

Lactobacillus-

Myconip Vaginal (Uni-Sankyo)

Nystanin-

Mycostatin Vag. (Sarabhai)

Chlorquinaldol-

Gynosen (S.P.P.L.)

Ketoconazole-

Phytoral Cream (B.B.)

Section- B

CHAPTER- 10

Endocrine System

Endocrine Glands

The endocrine system consists of a group of glands called "Endocrine Glands".

The endocrine glands are ductless glands, which pour their secretions directly into the blood stream and from where it is to be carried to the different parts of the body.

The Exocrine Glands viz.-the sweat glands, pour their secretions out through a duct.

The Pancreas, secretes both an exocrine and an endocrine secretions. These two types of secretions are formed in different types of cells present in the pancreas.

The hormones are the chemical messangers secreted from the endocrine glands. They are carried in the circulating blood to all parts of the body. Each hormone, however, can act on a specific group of cells or on a specific organ or organs only. These are known as target cells or target organs.

All endocrine glands have a chartacteristic structure consisting of secretory cells surrounded by connective tissue. The blood capillaries, lymphatics and nerves are situated in the connective tissue. The endocrine glands have a rich blood supply.

The endocrine gland's secretion is controlled by the

(i) Direct Regulation- e.g. insulin secretion, a high glucose level stimulates release of insulin, a low glucose level inhibits release of insulin.

(ii) Pituitary Feedback- The trophic hormones of pituitary, stimulate their target endocrine glands (e.g. adrenal cortex, ovary,etc) to secrete their hormones.

(iii) Hypothalamic Control- The hypothalamus produces some hormones which are carried out to pituitary gland and regulate the secretion of its trophic hormones.

The endocrine system regulates the activities of the body in order to maintain a state of equilibrium in the body with respect to various functions as well as the chemical composition of various body fluids and tissues.

Hormones

The Hormones are chemical substances synthesized and secreted by specialized cells and are carried in the blood stream and which act on specfic target tissues or organs.

Chemically hormones are proteins or steroids, or amines. The hormones are carried in the plasma partly in the free forms and partly bound to proteins.The free form of the hormone is the active form and when it is utilized by the body, the bound form of the hormone releases more free hormones for utilization.

The free hormones are metabolised in the liver either by chemical degradation or by conjugation. This metabolic degradation or conjugation makes the hormones less active or inactive.

Most of the hormones are insoluble in water. The conjugation makes them water soluble and thus facilitates their excretion by the kidneys.

The hormones are body's own drugs and act like a drug inrespect to their mechanism of action, metabolism and excretion from the body.

Types of Endocrine Glands

The important endocrine glands with definite endocrine functions are:

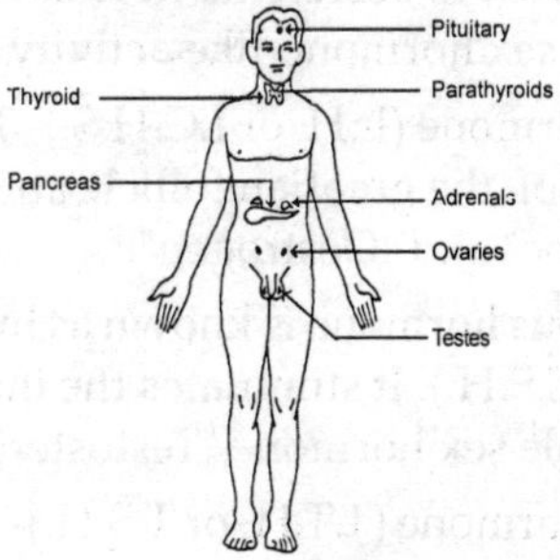

The Endocrine Glands

Fig.22

(A) Pituitary gland (B) Thyroid gland
(C) Parathyroid glands (D) Adrenal glands
(E) Ovary and Testes (F) Pancreas (Islets of Langerhans)
(G) Placenta & Corpus Luteum (During Pregnancy)

(A) Pituitary Gland- The pituitary consists of two lobes, viz. the anterior & the posterior lobes and controls all the endocrine glands.The pituitary is situated at the base of skull, connected to the hypothalamus (see fig-22). The pituitary is directly under the influence of hypothalamus.

(a) Anterior Pituitary- It consists of secretory cells surrounded by the connective tissues. It secretes different type of hormones, called "Trophic Hormones". A single trophic hormone stimulates only one target group of cells or organ.

The anterior pituitary lobe secretes the following hormones:

(i) Somatotrophin or Growth Hormone- The growth hormone stimulates tissue growth through its anabolic action and controls the growth of the body.

If it is produced in excess (Hypersecretion) during the childhood, it leads to excessive growth (Gigantism) and if it is secreted in excess after puberty leads to excessive enlargement of the hands, face and feet (Acromegaly). Diminished secretion on the other hand retards growth(Dwarfism).

(ii) Follicle Stimulating Hormone (FSH)- In the male , the FSH helps in the formation of spermatozoa in the testes. In the female, the FSH stimulates the development of the graafian follicle in the ovary.

(iii) Adrenocorticotrophic Hormone (ACTH)- The ACTH stimulate the adrenal cortex to secrete its hormones and a number of steroids with male sex hormone-like activity.

(iv) Luteinizing Hormone (L.H. or I.C.H.S.)- The L.H. leads to an increase in the size of the graafian follicle and controls the secretion of "Progesterone" and "Oestrogen".

In the male this hormone is known as interstitial cell stimulating hormone (I.C.S.H.). It stimulates the interstitial cells of the testes to secrete male sex hormone "Testosterone".

(v) Thyrotrophic Hormone (T.T.H. or T.S.H.)- It controls the activity of thyroid gland by stimulating the production of the thyroid hormone "Thyroxine".

(vi) Prolactin- In the female, it acts upon the Oestrogen & Progesterone primed mammary glands & initiates milk production and helps in the maintenance of Corpus Luteum & continued secretion of Progesterone during the pregnancy. In the male the action of Prolactin is not known.

The secretion of each trophic hormone is controlled by the blood concentration of the respective hormone of the target gland. It is also regulated by the appropriate releasing factor from the hypothalamus and stimuli of nervous origin.

(b) Posterior Pituitary- It consists of connective tissue, blood vessels and nerve fibres from the nuclei in hypothalamus. It is under nervous control and secrete two hormones

(i) Vasopressin or Antidiuretic Hormone (ADH)- It is elaborated and released by neurones of the hypothalamic nuclei. The hormone is migrated along the axons and stored in the posterior lobe of the pituitary gland.

The ADH exerts an antidiuretic effect by acting on the distal tubes of the kidney and helps in the reabsorption of water.

(ii) Oxytocin- It is also produced and relased by neurones of the hypothalamic nuclei and stored in the posterior lobe of the pituitary gland.

The oxytocin stimulates the contraction of the uterine smooth muscles and relaxes the lower part of the uterus (the cervix). This facilitates expulsion of the foetus during delivery and helps the contraction of uterus after the delivery (Involution).

The oxytocin also stimulates the contraction of the smooth muscles of the mammary glands leading to milk ejection (Let down).

The non pregnant uterus is not as sensitive to oxytocin as the pregnant uterus.

(B) Thyroid Gland- The Thyroid gland is located in the front of the neck and divided into two lobes situated on either side of the midline of the neck, which are connected by a small bridge.

The Thyroid gland's synthesize, store and secrete hormones,"Thyroxine"(T_4) & "Tri-iodothyronine" (T_3), under the control of the T.S.H. or T.T.H. from the anterior pituitary. It also secrets the hypocalcaemic hormone "Calcitonin".

These hormones (T_3 &T_4) are transported mostly bound to plasma proteins, and carried to the body cells. Iodine is a component of Thyroxine and therefore diet must provide iodine for the secretion of Thyroxine by the Thyroid gland.

The Thyroid hormones (T_3 &T_4) produce a calorigenic action and raise the basal metabolic rate (B.M.R.). It also increases carbohydrate and protein metabolism, increases hypolipidaemic effect, regulates the water & electrolyte balance and is essential for normal body growth, development and reproduction.

Its deficiency leads to "Cretinism" in young children and "Myoxedema" in adults. Where as excessive secretion of thyroid hormones gives rise to disease called "Thyrotoxicosis or Grave's disease" characterised by enlarged & swollen gland called " Goitre", which can also be due to deficiency of iodine in the diet or drinking water.

The Calcitonin main function is to produce "Hypocalcaemia" by inhibiting bone resorption and by promoting the urinary excretion of calcium and phosphorus. The release of Calcitonin is regulated by the ionized calcium concentration of the blood. Hypercalcaemia promotes the release of Calcitonin, and vice-versa.

(C) Parathyroid Glands- These are four small nodules situated in the neck, two on either side and embedded in the posterior surface of the thyroid gland.

The parathyroid glands secrete the hormone called,"Para-Thormone"(P.T.H.). The Parathromone's chief physiological role is the maintenance of "Calcium Homeostasis", which is an essential requirement for normal body function.

The parathormone promotes the absorption of calcium and phosphorus in the presence of Vitamin-D, from the intestine. It also promotes the resorption of the bone , releasing calcium into the blood. The PTH inhibits the renal tubular reabsorption of phosphate and decreases calcium clearance

The PTH release is mainly regulated by the calcium ion concentration in the blood . Release of PTH is stimulated by a fall and inhibited by a rise in the calcium ion concentration in the plasma.

Its overactivity leads to polyurea, polydipsia, renal calculi, subperiosteal bone resorption with hypercalcemia & hypercalciuria. On the other hand, its deficiency or removal of the Parathyroid gland results in a progressive fall in serum calcium levels, hypocalcaemia, tetany, convulsions and death.

(D) Adrenal Glands- The adrenals or suprarenal glands are two pyramid-shaped structure each lying at the top of its respective kidney. The adrenal glands are divided into two parts, the outer cortex and the central medulla. These two parts are functionally two distinct endocrine units.

(i) Adrenal Cortex- The cells of the adrenal cortex are arranged in three zones, and has no nerve supply.

The adrenal cortex secretes a large number of hormones. Chemically these hormones are steroids. The adrenal cortex secretes 30 hormones and are divided into three main groups:-

(I) Glucocorticoids- These are "Cortisol" (hydrocortisone) and "Corticosterone". They mainly effect carbohydrate metabolism and to a lesser extent protein and fat metabolism.

The Glucocorticoids have carbohydrate storing (storage of glycogen in the liver & muscles), antiallergic, antiinflammatory, protein catabolic (antianabolic effect) and cortieotrophin suppressing properties. It also inhibit the action of Vitamin-D in the intestine and reduces absorption of the calcium. It also increases gastric acid secretion.

(II) Mineralocorticoids- These are hormones which have an influence on metabolism. These are "Aldosterone" and "Deoxycorticosterone".

They act on renal tubules and produce sodium-retaining and potassium-depleting actions,and thereby influence salt and water metabolism.

An excess of Aldosterone leads to sodium retention, an increase in extracellular fluid volume and hypertension. Its deficiency leads to excessive loss of sodium, loss of extracellular fluid, lowering the blood volume and hypotension.

(III) Sex hormones - The "Androgen" (dehydroepiandrosterone) secreted has weaker masculinizing activity as compared to the Testosterone. The "Progesterone" and only a trace of "Oestrogen" (as Oestrone, Oestridiol and Oestriol) is secreted.

The adrenal sex hormones are of minor importance normally, but in adrenocortical hyperfunction they can cause the pathological symptoms.

The output of Glucocorticoids and Aldosterone may increase tenfold under the conditions of stress.

(ii) Adrenal Medulla- The adrenal medulla receives nerve supply from the ganglionic neurones of the sympathetic nervous system.

The adrenal medulla is composed of dark brown chromaffin cells which secrete "Catecholamines" (Adrenaline and Noradrenaline), which are mainly autonomic adrenergic agents.

The Adrenaline stimulates alpha and beta adrenergic receptors in various organs. Thus it raises the blood pressure, raises blood sugar, increases the heart rate & the cardiac output, etc. It is very useful in countering conditions of acute stress.

(E) Ovary and Testes- In both sexes, the gonads (ovaries & testes), besides their reproductive function, also possess an endocrine function.

(i) The Testes- The testes are two glandular bodies contained in the scrotum of the male. They form sperms and also the male sex hormones.

The male sex hormones or "Androgens" are mainly secreted by the testes and to a lesser extent by the adrenal cortex (androstenedione) and the ovary (dehydro- epiandrosterone). The most potent natural androgen is "Testosterone" and is secreted by the testicular interstitial cells of Leydig.

At puberty, the FSH stimulates the metabolic activity of the Sertoli cells in the seminiferous tubules, and promotes spermatogenesis. The ICSH promotes the development of the interstitial cells, which synthesize and secrete "Testosterone". The secretion is regulated by a hypothalamic - pituitary servomechanism.

The Testosterone brings about the development of secondary sex characters, viz. growth of facial & body hair, deep voice, penile growth, development of muscle tissue, development of prostate gland & seminal vesicles and development of sex drive. It also support spermatogenesis and regulate secretion of gonadotrophins. These characteristics are maintained after puberty by the continued secretion of Testosterone.

The testes also produce small amount of Oestrogen (female

sex hormone), but the Testosterone activity predominates. The active form of Testosterone is 5 alpha dihydrotestosterone.

(ii) The Ovaries- The ovaries are two in number, are small almond sized glands situated in the lower abdomen. The ovaries produce two female sex hormones, Oestrogen and Progesterone. The small amount of androgens are also secreted by the adrenal cortex in the females, but the female sex hormones activity predominate. In the ovaries Oestrogen are secreted by the Graafian Follicle, and Progesterone is secreted by the Corpus Luteum.

The Oestrogen and Progesterone regulate the menstrual cycle in women. The female sex hormones are synthesized in the ovaries (mainly), adrenals, placenta and testes. The anterior pituitary controls the secretion of ovarian hormones by the feed back machanism.

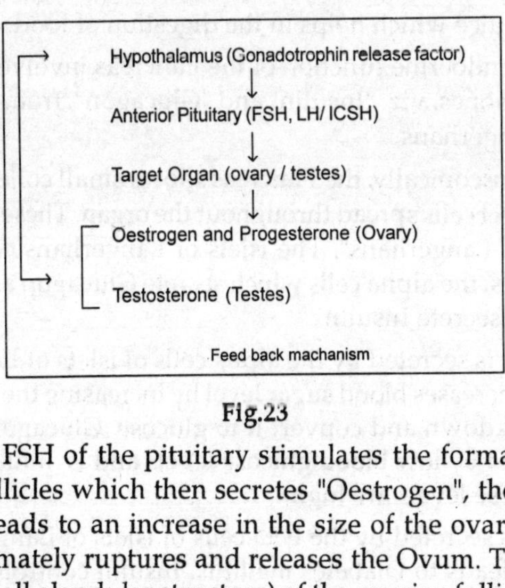

Fig.23

The FSH of the pituitary stimulates the formation of the ovarian follicles which then secretes "Oestrogen", the LH of the pituitary leads to an increase in the size of the ovarian follicle, which ultimately ruptures and releases the Ovum. The residual mass (a small glandular structure) of the ovarian follicle after the expulsion of ovum is known as "Corpus Luteum", which secretes Progesterone.

The main natural Oestrogens produced by the women are Oestradiol, Oestriol and Oestrone. The Oestrogen brings about the development of the female secondary sexual characteristics, viz. development of breast, distribution of body hair, characteristic distribution of body fat, growth of uterus & vagina.

It also prepares the endometrium for Progestogen action & for spermatozoal transport and induces mild anabolism.

The Progesterone is a steroid derivative of Pregnane, is the main natural Progestogen, besides 17 - alpha hydroxyprogesterone, 20 - alpha - hydroxyprogesterone are also natural Progestogens. The Progesterone brings about proliferation of glands in the endometrium (secretory phase), it prepares uterus to receive the embryo, maintains uterus during pregnancy, stimulates the growth of mammary glands (but suppresses milk secretion), induces mild catabolic effect. The female sex hormones also regulate the secretion of gonadotrophins.

(F) Pancreas- Pancreas is a gland situated horizantly below and behind the stomach. It is a mixed gland and performs both exocrine and endocrine functions.

The exocrine function of the Pancreas involves secretion of pancreatic juice which helps in the digestion of food.

The endocrine function of the Pancreas involves secretion of two hormones, viz. "Insulin" and "Glucagon", from the cells of islets of Langerhans.

Microscopically, the Pancreas shows small collection or islets of distinct cells spread throughout the organ. These are known as "Islets of Langerhans". The islets of Langerhans contain two types of cells; the alpha cells which secrete Glucagon and the beta cells which secrete Insulin.

Glucagon- It is secreted by the alpha cells of islets of Langerhans. Glucagon increases blood sugar level by increasing the stored glycogen breakdown and convert it to glucose. Glucagon secretion is stimulated by low blood glucose levels and is inhibited when blood glucose levels are high.

Insulin- It is secreted by the beta cells of islets of Langerhans. Its deficiency leads to Diabetes mellitus. Insulin controls the blood sugar level and mantains it within its normal range.

The insulin is a polypeptide, the normal Pancreas contains about 200 units of insulin and normally man secretes about 50 units of insulin daily. Insulin reduces blood sugar level by the following mechanisms

(a) Membrane effects- Increased glucose, amino acid, fatty acid transport and cellular uptake of K+ and Mg ++.

(b) Intracelluar effects

(i) Increased Protein, RNA & DNA synthesis

(ii) Depress gluconeogenesis (conversion of fats & proteins to glucose)

(iii) Stimulation of glycogen synthesis.

(iv) Increased Lipogenesis.

(v) Increase oxidation of glucose in the tissues.

(vi) Break down of glycogen to glucose decreased.

When the blood glucose level is low, the beta cells are not stimulated & secretion of insulin is discontinued.

(G) Placenta and Corpus Luteum- Both of them secrete female sex hormones, in case fertilization takes place and the ovum gets implanted into the endometrium of the uterus (Pregnancy). The Corpus Luteum secretes Oestrogen and Progesterone up to 99th day and 100th day onward of pregnancy the placenta takes over the secretion of female sex hormones from the Corpus Luteum.

Table - 3 Endocrine Glands and their Hormones

S.No.	EndocrineGland	Hormone
1.	Pituitary Gland	(i) Somatotrophin or Growth hormone.
	(a) Anterior lobe	(ii) ACTH (Adrenocorticotrophic hormone).
		(iii) FSH (Follicle stimulating hormone).
		(iv) Luteinizing hormone LH in female, ICSH in male
		(v) TSH/TTH (Thryrotrophic hormone)
		(vi) Prolactin
	(b) Posterior lobe	(i) ADH (Antidiuretic hormone or Vasopressin).
		(ii) Oxytocin
2.	Thyroid Gland	(i) Thyroxine
		(ii) Calcitonin
3.	Parathyroid Glands	(i) PTH (Parathormone hormone)
4.	Adrenal Glands	
	(a) Cortex	(i) Glucocorticoids (Cortisol, Corticosterone)
		(ii) Mineralocorticoids (Aldosterone, Deoxycorticosterone)

		(iii) Sex hormones - Androgen (week Testosterone) - Progesterone - Oestrogen
	(b) Medulla	(i) Adrenaline (ii) Noradrenaline
5.	Testes	(i) Androgens (Testosterone) (ii) Oestrogen (V. small amount)
6.	Ovaries	(i) Oestrogen (ii) Progesterone
7.	Pancreas (Islets of Langerhans) (a) Alpha cells (b) Beta cells	 (i) Glucagon (i) Insulin

Clinical Aspects

Acromegly- Excessive enlargement of the hands, face and feet, occuring in adult due to excess secretion of the growth hormone.

Adrenal hyperplasia- Exessive formation of cells of adrenal glands.

Cretinism- It is a congenital thyroid deficiency disorder, resulting in a dull-looking child (underdeveloped mently & physically).

Cushing's disease- It occurs rarely due to excessive ACTH & Glucocorticoids (hydrocortisone) secretion, characterized by virilism, obesity, hyperglycaemia, hypertension and glycosuria mainly in females.

Diabetes insipidus- It is a congenital or following injury / infecton disease of the posterior gland or its adnexa, characterized by dehydration, polyuria, polydipsia, pale colour urine with low specific gravity.

Diabetes millitus- It is a hereditary disorder with metabolic & vascular derangements, which are possibly interrelated. It is characterized by -

(i) Hyperglycaemia with a deranged secretion of Insulin & possibly Glucagon.

(ii) Thickening of the basement membranes of capillaries throughout the body.

(iii) Complications involving the glomerulus, retina and peripheral nervous system, leading to renal failure, blindness and neuropathy.

The main use of insulin is in the treatment of Diabetes mellitus as a replacement therapy in insulin dependent Diabetes mellitus (IDDM). The NIDDM means non insulin dependent Diabetes mellitus. In diabetic coma, the patient become unconscious due to ketoacidosis.

Dwarfism- Retarted growth due to diminished secretion of the Growth hormone.

Gigantism- Hypersecretion of the growth hormone during the childhood, leads to excessive growth.

Glycosuria- The presence of sugar in the urine.

Goitre- It is an enlargement of Thyroid gland due to excessive secretion of thyroid hormones.

Hypercalciuria- Excessive calcium excretion in the urine.

Hyperglycaemia- Excessive sugar in the blood.

Hyperinsulinism- Excessive insulin from the pancreatic islets lowering the blood sugar, which can leads to intermittent of continuous loss of consciousness, with or without convulsions.

Hyperkalaemia- Excessive potassium in the blood.

Hyperparathyroidism- Increase in the serum calcium levels due to overaction of the Parathyroid glands.

Hypocalcaemia- Decreased calcium concentration in the blood.

Hypoglycaemia- Decreased blood sugar charcterised by anxiety, excitement, perspiration, delirium or coma.

Hypokalaemia- Abnormally low potassium level of the blood.

Hypoparathyroidism- Decreased in the serum calcium levels due to underaction of the Parathyroid glands (Causing tetany).

Hypopituitarism- A disorder mainly occurs due to anterior lobe of Pituitary gland insuffeciency.

Myxoedema- It is a clinical syndrom of hypothyrioidism, may leads to bradycardia, swelling of face & limbs, low temperature, dryskin, patient becomes slow in movement and dull mentally.

Shock- The circulatory distrubance produced by severe illness or injury and due to reduction in blood volume, may leads to hypotension, restlessness, thirst & a cold clammy skin.

Simmond's disease- In this the patient becomes emaciated with sparse & grey hairs, undully wrinkled, slow pulse & hypotension. Previously also called as Panhypopituitarism.

Thyroiditis- Inflammation of the Thyroid gland.

Thyrotoxicosis- It is a condition due to excessive production of the Thyroxine chracterized by- anxiety, tachycardia, sweating, increased appetite with weight loss and a fine tremor of the outstretched hands & prominence of the eyes.

Applied Medicines

(1) Corticosteroids and related drugs- The adrenal corticosteroid drugs are amongst the most widely empolyed of all therapeutic agents. They sometimes exert dramatic effects which helps the patient to tide over the critical stage of acute illness. They only offer a symptomatic relief and its prolonged use necessarily leads to adverse effects.

The adrenocorticosteroid are used either in physiological dose as a replacement therapy to correct a deficiency (e.g. hypopituitarism) or in pharmacologic doses to treat inflammatory disorders, allergic states, collagen disorders, ophthalmic diseases, acute infectious diseases, neoplastic diseases and several other diseases.

Hydrocortisone-

Efcorlin Inj. (Glaxo), Wycort Inj. (Wyeth)

Dexamethasone-

Decdan (Merind), Dexona (Cadila H.C.), Wymesone (Wyeth)

Fluticasone-

Flutivate (Glaxo), Zoflut (Cipla)

Betamethasone-

Betnesol (Glaxo), Celestone (Fluford), Stemin (Indswift), Walacort (Wallace)

Prednisolone-

Deltacortril (Pfizer), Wysolone (Wyeth),Omnacortil (Macleods) Depo-Medrol Inj. (Upjohn), Predicort (Macmillon)

Triamcinolone-

Comcort (Comed), Ledercort (Wyeth), Pericort (Themis)

(2) Hypo And Hyperglycaemics-

(i) Sulphonylureas- They are chemically related to sulphonamides, but have no antibacterial activity. The sulphonylureas stimulate the beta-cell islet tissue to secrete insulin.

Chlorpropamide-

Chlorformin (Cadila), Copamide (Deys), Diabinese (Pfizer)

Tolbutamide-

Rastinon (Hoechst)

Gliclazide-

Diamicron (Serdia), Glycigon (Aristo), Glizid (Panacea)

Glibenclamide-

Daonil (Hoechst), Euglucon (Nicholas), Glucosafe (Sun), Glibet (C.F.L.)

Glipizide -

Glynase (USV), M-Diab (Upjohn), Glide (Franco)

(ii) Biguanides- They stimulate the peripheral utilization of glucose and reduce the intestinal absorption of glucose.

Phenformin-

DBI (USV)

Metformin-

Gluformin (Nicholas), Glycomet (USV), Bigomet (Gentica), Diamet (Bal Ph.), Glumet (Cipla)

(iii) Glucagon- It mobilises glycogen stored in the liver. Inj. Glucagon (Torrent)

(iv) Insulin- It is a water soluble polypeptide, use mainly as a replacement therapy in the treatment of Diabetes mellitus. These preparations contain either animal or human insulin.

Inj. Insulins (Knoll), Insulins Zinc sus. (Lente).

Inj. ILetin-L, ILetin-N, ILetin-R (Eli Lilly),

Inj. Actrapid, Actrapid MC, Mixtard, Insulatard (Knoll)

Inj. Rapidica, Rapimix, Zinulin (Sarabhai).

Inj. Huminsulin, Huminsulin-L, Huminsulin-N,

Huminsulin-R, Huminsulin-UL (Eli Lilly),

Inj. Human Rapidica, Human Rapimix,

Human Zinulin (Sarabhai), Inj. Actraphane HM,

Human Actrapid, Human Mixtard, Human Insulatard (Knoll)

(3) Thyroid And Antithyroid Drugs- The thyroid drugs increase the metabolic rate with a subsequent increase in catabolism.

The antithyroid drugs inhibit formation of thyroid hormones in the thyroid gland.

Thyroxine-

Proloid (Parke Davis), Roxin (Cadila H.C.), Eltroxin (Glaxo)

Iodine-

Collosol Iodine (Duphar)

Carbimazole-

Neomercazole (Nicholas), Thyrozole (Cadila Ph.)

(4) Anabolics-

Refer to Chapter -5 (Section B)

(5) Androgenic Steroids, Fertility Agents And Trophic Hormones - Refer to Chapter -9 (Section B)

(6) Other Hormones-

Somatostatin-

Stilamin (Serum Institute), Sandostatin (Novartis)

Epoietin (Erythropoietin)-

Eprex (Ethnor), Zyrop (Cadila H.C.)

Salmon Calcitonin-

Calsynar (Rhone-Poulenc)

Somatrophin (Growth Hormone)-

Genotropin (Pharmacia), Saizen (Serum)

Vasopressin-

Petresin (Shree Ganesh)

Desmopressin-

D-Void (Sun)

Section- B

CHAPTER- 11

Organs of Special Senses

The special sense organs include skin, eyes, ears, nose and tongue. These organs provide man with information about his environments so that he can formulate appropriate responses.

The Skin

The skin protects from the external enviornments. The outer layer of skin is relatively resistant to wear & tear, and is water repellant & prevents seepage of water in it. As a sense organ it conveys temperature, pressure, pain and touch to the brain and also helps in the regulation of our body temperature, which is under the control of hypothalamus. The skin serves as a depot of fats as well as an insulating layer against cold. The skin also helps to form Vitamin-D_3 (Cholecalciferol) under the influence of the sun's ultraviolet rays.

As shown in fig.-24, the skin consists of two layers, the outerone called "Epidermis" and thick innerone called "Dermis" (Corium). Beneath the dermis is the subcutaneous adipose tissue or fat.

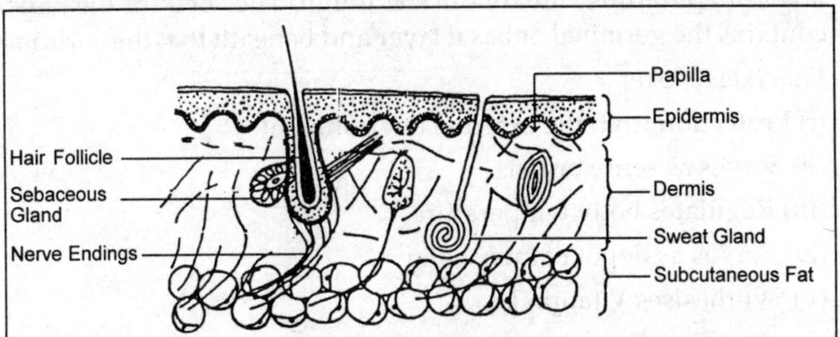

Section of Skin

Fig.24

The epidermis is a stratified squamous epithelium, consisting of layers. The outermost is composed of the protein known as "Keratin" derived from dead cells. The basal one contains cells known as "Melanocytes", which synthesise and store the pigment "Melanin", which impart colour to the skin. The nutritional material is supplied through the tissue fluid present in dermis, as blood vessels are not present in epidermis.

The dermis is composed of fibro-elastic tissue. It is richly supplied with blood vessels and nerves.The dermis also cantains hair follicles, sweatglands and sebaceous glands. Histamine containing cell (mast cells) are found in dermis close to the blood vessels; during allergic reactions (e.g.urticaria) they release histamine. The projections of dermis present towards the epidermis are called "Papillae". The free sensory nerve endings are found near the epidermis and around the base of hair follicles, and other sensory nerve endings are incorporated in specialised structures the "Pacinian Corpuscles", which are senstive to pressure & the "Meissner's Corpuscles", which are sensitive to touch.

The sweat glands are coiled glands situated in dermis & open on the surface of skin. They secrete "Sweat" (about 500 ml. per day), which contains water, sodium, chloride & potassium.

The hair follicles are deep invaginations of the epidermis and shafts of hair grow from their floor.

The sebaceous glands open into the sides of hair follicles and secrete "Sebum" (oily substance) that lubricates the skin surface, the hair shaft and imparts shine to the hair.

The nails corrospond structurally to the second or clear layer of epidermis and are thick & tough. The "Bed" of the nails contains the germinal or basal layer and beneath that the corium.

Functions of Skin

(i) Protection from the external environment.

(ii) Serves as sense organ.

(iii) Regulates body temperature.

(iv) Serves as depot of fats; water.

(v) Synthesises Vitamin D_3.

Causes of Skin Diseases

(i) Infections (Bacterial, Fungal, Viral, Parasitic)

(ii) Allergy
(iii) Trauma (Burns)
(iv) Heredity
(v) Auto-immune mechanism
(vi) Neoplasms

The Eye

Eyes are the organs of sight. Apart from enabling a person to see the objects, it also help him get a sense of position and thus facilitate maintenance of balance.

The "Eye Ball" is located in a bony cave called, the "Orbit" and protected in front by the "Eyelids". The eyeball is nearly spherical in shape and has three coats or layers, the outer one is "Sclera", the middle one is "Choroid" and the inner one is "Retina". The movements of the eyeball are brought about by a set of six muscles attached to it & the orbit.

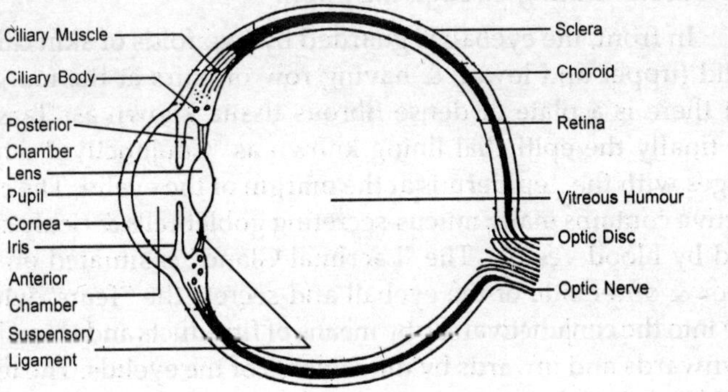

Section of Eye Ball

Fig.-25

The sclera or sclerotic is consisting of dense fibrous tissue and is opaque, it can be seen in front as white of the eye. The dome-shaped, circular, transparent structure at the front of the eyeball is known as "Cornea" and at the periphery it merges with the sclera, and the junction is known as "Limbus". The cornea has no blood vessels, and covered outside by stratified epithelium & inside by a simple epithelium. At its back, the sclera is pierced by the optic nerve and the optic blood vessels.

The choroid is pigmented and contains blood vessels. It is continued towards the front with the "Ciliary Body", which contains the "Ciliary Muscle". Anteriorly, the ciliary body is continuous with the "Iris". The aperture of iris is known as the "Pupil". The transparent & avascular, "Lens" is suspended behind the iris with the help of a fibrous ring known as the "Suspensory Ligament".

The retina covers only the rear five-sixths of the eyeball. The retina is a thin membrane containing light-sensitive structures, the "Rods" & the "Cones", from which arise the sensory fibres of the optic nerve.These fibres converge at the "Optic Disc", the point at which the optic nerve emerges from the eyeball.

The interior of the eyeball is divided into two compartments, one behind the lens & contains a transparent, jelly-like substance known as "Vitreous Humour" and one in front of the lens & contains tissue fluid known as "Aqueous Humour". The iris divides the chamber containing aqueous humour into two parts viz. "Anterior Chamber" and "Posterior Chamber";and these two communicating through the pupil.

In front, the eyeball is guarded by two folds of skin called eyelid (upper and lower, & having row of hairs at the margin) next there is a plate of dense fibrous tissue known as "Tarsus" and finally the epithelial lining known as "Conjunctiva" which merges with the epidermis at the margin of the eyelid. The conjunctiva contains many mucus-secreting goblet cells & richly supplied by blood vessels. The "Lacrimal Gland" is situated on the upper & outer side of the eyeball and secrets the "Tears" which flow into the conjunctival sac by means of fine ducts and is washed downwards and inwards by movements of the eyelids. The tears are thin, watery secretion also contain an enzyme called lysozyme and keep the conjunctiva moist & helps wash away any dust & foreign particles that may settle on it.

Functions of the Eye

(i) Vision, enabling us to see objects.

(ii) Helps in the maintenance of balance.

The Ear

It is basically an organ for the perception of sound. The ear consists of three sections:

(i) External ear,

(ii) Middle ear,

(iii) Internal ear.

The external ear is consisting of funnel -like structure the "Pinna" & the external ear canal. The pinna is made up of elastic cartilage and coverd with skin, which is extended up to external ear canal.

The middle ear or "Tympanum" is a chamber situated between external & internal ear. It is lined by ciliated epithelium and communicates with pharynx via "Eustachean Tube". The "Ear Drum" or "Tympanic Membrane" separates the middle ear from the external ear. The ear drum is lined by epidermis on the outerside and by ciliated epithelium on the innerside. The ear drum is connected to the internal ear by a link of three little bones called "Auditory Ossicles" (outer- 'malleus', middle-'incus' and inner-'stapes'), by which magnify vibrations are transmitted to the internal ear.

The internal ear is a bony structure consisting of a "Vestibule", a set of three "Semicircular Canals" and a spiral "Cochlea" (an organ of hearing). The eighth cranial or "Auditory Nerve" arises from the internal ear.

Functions of the Ear

(i) Hearing.

(ii) Organ for the sense of position and movement that is essential to the maintenance of balance.

The Nose

The nasal cavity is situated between the skull cavity above and the oral cavity below. It is divided lengthwise into two halves by means of a partition called the "Nasal Septum". Each half of the nasal cavity is open in front to the exterior called the "Nostrils" and behind it opens into the nasopharynx. Inside, these nostrils are rich in hair follicles. The lateral wall of the nasal cavity have three shelf like projections called "Conchae" or "Turbinate" (superior, middle & inferior), running from the front towards the rear. Each conchae forms a tunnel like passage called "Meatuses" (superior, middle & inferior), running along the length of the lateral wall.

The epithelial lining covering the upper 10 m.m. of the nasal cavity is known as "Olfactory epithelium". It contains specialised nerve cells known as "Olfactory Cells", whose dendrites are the smell - sensitive nerve endings and whose axons form the sensory fibres of the olfactory nerves. The epithelium also contains mucous glands in whose secretion, volatile substances dissolve and then stimulate the olfactory nerve endings. The fibres of the olfactory cells pass into the skull through a perforated plate of bone in the roof of the nasal cavity and join to form the "Olfactory Nerve".

Functions of the Nose

1. It serve as the organ of the sense of smell.
2. Acts as resonator of the nasal sounds of speech.
3. Helps the inhaled air to enter in the lungs as moist, warm & free of dust, and foreign particles.

The Tongue

The tongue is an organ of taste. The core of the tongue is formed by voluntary muscle tissue, the surface being madeup of stratified squamous epithelium. On the upper surface, the epithelium has minute projections called "Papillae" of various sizes and shapes. Embedded in these papillae are the taste buds (Organs of taste). The taste sensitive cells or "Gustatory Cells" open in each taste bud by means of small pore.

The sensory fibres, which carry taste sensation arise from the gustatory cells. The sensation of taste is carried from the tongue by two cranial nerves, the facial nerve & the glossopharyngeal nerve. The motor nerve fibres to the tongue muscles are supplied through the hypoglossal nerve. The tip of tongue is more sensitive to sweet taste, the sides to sour taste, the upper surface to salty taste and the rear portion to bitter taste.

Functions of the Tongue

1. To create a sensation of taste.
2. Forms an important part of the speech mechanism.
3. Aids the chewing & swallowing of food.

Clinical Aspects

(i) Skin-

Allergy- An allergy is a sensitivity to a substance which does not normally cause people any discomfort or harm. Allergies are a reaction to antigen-antibody. Allergies can be caused by milk, egg, fish, insect bites, animal hair, chemicals, artificial Jewellery, dustmites, heat, cold & variety of natural & artificial substances.

Alopecia- Baldness or loss of hair.

Acne Vulgaris- A skin condition common in adolescence, characterised by black heads with a papular & pustular eruption of the pilosebaceous follicles. Usual sites are the face, neck, upper part of chest & back.

Balanitis- Inflammation of the glans penis & prepuce.

Boils (Furncles)- Acute inflammatory conditions surrounding the hair follicles, caused due to Staphylococcus aureus.

Burn- A lesion of the tissue due to flame, dry heat, chemicals, electricity, or radiation.

Candidiasis- A disease caused by infection with species of Candida. (e.g. C. vulvitis, Fungal nappy rashes, C. paronychia).

Chilblain- Congestion, swelling, severe itching & burning sensation in reaction to cold.

Dermatitis- Inflammation of the skin caused due to various reasons (viz. dust, soaps, chemicals, liquid or allergens), with erythema, itching, burning.

Eczema- It is the inflammation & necrosis of the epidermis with exudation of fluid from the dermis. It is a hypersensitive reaction to an irritant.

Epidermophytosis- Infection of the skin & nail caused by fungi of genus Epidermophyton.

Erythema- Reddening of the skin-erythematous

Folliculitis- Inflammation of follicles or boils, most often due to Staphylococcal infections.

Herpes- A vasicular eruption caused due to a virus infection, caused by-

> **H. simplex-** Appearance of blisters around the mouth,
>
> **H.zoster-** Appearance of vesicles along the distribution of the nerves involved, with severe pain.

Hyperkeratosis- Hypertrophy of the cornea or the horny layer of the skin.

Hypertrichosis- Excessive growth of hair.

Ichthyosis- A congenital condition of the skin which is dry & scaly.

Impetigo- An inflammatory pustular disease caused by Staphylococcus & Streptococcus.

Leucoderma- The presence of white, non-pigmented patches.

Otitis Externa- Inflammation of the skin of the external auditory canal.

Paronychia- Supporative inflammation around a finger - nail.

Pediculosis- Infestation with a genus of parasitic insects (lice)

Pityriasis- Scaly eruption of the skin (e.g. P. capitis or dandruff).

Pruritus- Allergic reaction may cause stimulation of sensory nerves and itching(e.g. - P. ani, P. vulvae)

Pyoderma- Chronic infection of the skin caused by micro-organism leading to pus formation.

Ringworm- A contagious infection of the skin caused by a fungus and characterised by circular scaly patches.

Scabies- A highly contagious parasitic skin disease caused by the itch mite.

Sycosis barbai- A pustular folliculitis of the beard area in men.

Tinea- A contagious fungal infection of the skin. Described as per the affected parts of the body viz. T. pedis (Foot), T. capitis (Head), T. corporis (Body), T. cruris. (Perineum & Perinial region), T. barbae (Beard in men), T. ungnium (Nail).

Urticaria- An allergic skin disorder characterized by exudation of fluid from blood vessels, leading to formation of flat, raised swelling.

(2) Eye & Ear

Blepharitis- Inflammation of the eyelid, particularly the edges.

Cataract- A condition where the lens becomes opaque owing to degenerative change. It may be senile, congenital, traumatic or due to diabetes mellitus. It is of two types, hard cataract and soft cataract.

Conjunctivitis- Inflammation of the conjunctiva due to infection/ injury.

Dacrocystitis- Inflammation of the tear sac.

Epiphora- Pathological overflow of tears.

Glaucoma- A condition where the intraocular pressure is raised. It causes intense pain.

Hypermetropia- Inability to see near objects clearly.

Iridocyclitis- Inflammation of the iris & ciliary body.

Iritis- Inflammation of the iris.

Keratitis- Inflammation of the cornea.

Keratocojunctivitis- Inflammation of the cornea & conjunctiva.

Keratoiritis- Inflammation of the cornea and iris.

Keratomalacia- Softening of the cornea, ulceration may occur, caused by Vitamin-A deficiency.

Labyrinthithis- Inflammation of the internal ear.

Mastoiditis- Infection of mastoid bone behind the ear. It is a very painful condition.

Menier's disease- Distention of membranous labyrinth of middle ear from excess fluid. It is a non-infective condition accompanied with giddiness.

Myopia- Inability to see distant objects clearly.

Otitis Externa- Inflammation of the skin of the external auditory canal caused due to bacterial infection, fungus.

Otitis Media- Inflammation of the middle ear, causes pain & fever.

Otomycosis- A fungal infection of the external auditory meatus.

Otorrhoea- A discharge from the external auditory meatus.

Otosclerosis- Formation of new bone, affecting the labyrinth of the inner ear. A common cause of progressive deafness.

Photo-Phobia- Inability to expose the eyes to light.

Presbyopia- In old age the lens gradually loses its elasticity resulting long sightedness.

Retinitis- Inflammation of the retina.

Scleritis- Inflammation of the outer layer of eye.

Stye- An abscess in the follicle of an eyelash.

Trachoma- It is contagious inflammation caused by "Bedsonia" affecting conjunctiva, cornea and eyelids.

Uveitis- Inflammation of the uvea (the pigmented part of eye).

(3) Nose & Tongue

Anosmia- Inability to smell.

Glossitis- Inflammation of the tongue, due to infection or deficiency of certain Vitamins.

Nasopharyngitis- Inflammation of the nasopharynx.

Rhinitis- Inflammation of the nasal mucous membrane.

Rhinorrhoea- Nasal discharge.

Sneezing- The emitting of air suddenly with explosive sound from the nose, mainly due to allergen.

Stammering- A psychological disoders of speech due to improper co-ordination of muscles.

Applied Medicines

Besides Antibiotics, Nutrients and N.S.A.I.D's where requried following are some medicines used in

(1) Skin

(i) Antiallergic- These drugs prevent or lessen allergy by competitively inhibiting H_1 receptors. Chlorpheniramine

Piriton (Glaxo), Polaramine (Fulford).

Pheniramine Maleate-

Avil (Hoechst).

Diphenhydramine-

Benadryl (Parke-Davis)

Mebhydrolin Napadisylate-

Incidal (Bayer)

Dimethindene Maleate-

Foristal (Novartis)

Astemizole-

Alerzole (Themis Pharma), Astelong (Torrent), Stemiz (Cadila H.C.)

Terfenadine-

Terfed (Protec), Trexyl (Ranbaxy), Zoter (Cadila Ph.), Terfax (Kopran)

Clemastine-

Tavegyl (Novartis), Tavist (Wander)

Cetrizine-

Alday (SOL), Alerid (Cipla), Citrazan (Mac), Zyncet (Unichem), CZ-3 (Lupin)

Loratidine-

Loridin (Cadila H.C.), Lorfast (La-Sante)

Azatadine Maleate-

Zadine (Fulford)

Hydroxyzine-

Atarax (Uni-Ucb)

Fexofenadine-

Allegra (Hoechst), Altiva (Ranbaxy)

(ii) Topical Antifungals- These drugs distorys the fungi by causing leakage of their cellular contents used in Candidal infections, Ringworm (Tinea), Athlete's foot, etc.

Tolnaftate-

Tinaderm (Fulford), Tinavate (Dabur)

Quiniodochlor-

Dermo-Quinol (East India), Vioform (Novartis)

Miconazole-

Daktarin (Ethnor), Zole (Rexcel), Candistat (Merck)

Clotrimazole-

Canesten (Bayer), Imidil (Lyka), Statum (Croslands), Surfaz (Franco), Candid (Glenmark), Mycoban (Perch)

Ciclopirox Olamine-

Batrafen (Roussel), Laprox-F (Lyka)

Ketoconazole-

Funginoc (Torrent), Nizral (Ethnor), Phytoral (B & B)

(iii) Topical Anti-Parasitics- These drugs prevent or destroy parasites. Used commonly in Scabies, Pediculosis etc.

Gammabenzene Hexachloride-

Emscab (M.M.Lab.), Lorexane (ICI), Scabex (Indoco), Scarab (Aristo), Ultrascab (Perch), Nit-N- Mite (Makers)

Benzyl Benzoate-

Ascabiol (Rhone-Poulenc), Scabindon (Indon)

Crotamiton-

Crotorax (S.P.P.L.)

Permethrin-

Perlice & Permite (Croslands)

(iv) Topical anti-infectives- These preparations includes antibiotic, antiseptics and antiviral agents.

Nitrofurazone-

Furacin (S.B.)

Neomycin-

Neosporin (Wellcome)

Gentamycin-

Merigenta (Mercury), Lyramycin (Lyka)

Framycetin-

Soframycin(Roussel)

Sisomicin-

Ensamycin (Fulford)

Silver Sulphadiazine-

Dibact (Sigma), Silverex (Croslands), Alorex (Pure) Silver Sulphadiazine (Indon & Duphar)

Fusidic Acid-

Fucidin (Crosslands), Fusiderm (Indipharma)

Cetrimide-

Cetavolon (ICI), Endruff (Nulife)

Chloroxylenol-

Dettol (RCI), Iteol-3 (Astro-IDL)

Povidone Iodine-

Betadine (Win-Medicare), Wokadine (Wockhardt)

Acyclovir-

Acivir (Cipla), Cyclovir (Cadila H.C.), Herpex Cream (Torrent)

(V) Topical Steroids- These drugs exerts anti-inflammatory, anti-allergic, anti-proliferative, anti-pruritic and anti-eczematous actions. Used commonly in eczema, psoriasis, etc.

Hydrocortisone-

Cortoquinol (East India), Wycort (Wyeth), Crotorax HC(SG Pharma)

Betamethasone-

Betamil (Merck), Betnovate (Glaxo), Diprovate (Croslands)

Beclomethasone-

Beclate (Cipla), Derbec (Alkem), Zovate (Allenburys)

Clobetasol-

Clobetamil (Merck), Clobispan (Merind), Tenovate (Glaxo)

Triamcinolone-

Ledercort (Cyanamid), Cortrima (Nulife)

Clobetasone-

Eumosone (Glaxo)

Dexamethasone-

Millicortenol (Novartis), Sofradex (Roussel)

Fluocinolone-

Alcort (Alembic), Flucort (Lyka), Supricort (Glenmark)

Clostebol-

Clostagen (Elder), Trofodermin (Upjohn)

(VI) Topical Preparations for Mixed Infections-

Betnovate-N, Betnovate-C (Glaxo),Cloben, Cloben-G (Indoco), Cortoquinol (East India), Multicorten-Vioform (Novartis), Lobate-G, Lobate -M (Nicholas), Tenovate-G, Tenovate-M(Glaxo), Coraryl-H (FDC), Betamil-M, Betamil GM (Merck), Quiss (Jagson pal), Gentalence-C (Crossland), Sigmaderm (Sigma), Quadriderm (Fulford), Superderm (Twilight), Candiderma (Glenmark), Zole-F (Rexcel).

(VII) Miscellaneous Topical Preparations-

Antiacne-

Persol Gel (Wallace), Pernox Gel (CFL Pharma), Acnex (Unisearch), Acnesol (Systopic), Retino-A (Ethnor), Eskamel (S.B.), Acniderm (Abbott)

Anti-thrombotics-

Beparine (B.E.), Thrombophob (German Remedies)

Antipsoriatics-

Manaderm (Wyeth), Neosoralen (Mac), Mycoderm (F.D.C.) Daivonex (Croslands), Derobin (Glaxo).

Drugs for Baldness-

Multigain (Torrent), Hebald (Intas), Mintop (DRL)

Pigmentation Disorders-

Melanocyl (Franco-Indain), Macsoralen (Mac)

Anti-Seborrheics-

Dermogard (Indipharma), Pragmatar (S.B.), Selsun (Abbott)

(2) Eye

(i) Ocular Anti-infectives- These preparations include antibacterials, anti fungals & Antiviral agents.

Oxytetracycline-

Oint. Oxytetracycline (Pfizer)

Sulphacetamide-

Albucid Nicholas), Locula (East India), Setride (Merind)

Chloramphenicol-

Enteromycetin (Dey's), Paraxin (Nicholas), Vanmycetin (FDC)

Gentamicin-

Genticyn (Nicholas), Gentamicin (Fulford), Merigenta (Mercury), Gentasporin (PCI)

Ciprofloxacin-

Cifran Eye (Ranbaxy), Ciplox (Cipla), Zoxan (FDC), Ciprobid E/E (Cadila H.C.), Zoptic (Mejda), Alcipro (Alkem)

Norfloxacin-

Norbactin Eye (Ranbaxy), Norbid E/E (Alembic), Norflox (Cipla)

Pefloxacin-

Proflox (Protec)

Tobramycin-

Tobacin (Aristo), Tobazon (Bell Pharma)

Soframycin-

Soframycin (Roussel)

Polymyxin-B-

Andresporin (Andre), Neosporin Eye (Wellcome), Pychlor (Mac), Ocupol (Centaur)

Miconazole-

Micoptic (FDC)

Fluconazole-

Syscan (Torrent), Zocon (F.D.C.)

Natamycin-

Pimafucin (Elder)

Acyclovir-

Acivir (Cipla), Herpex Optha. (Torrent), Ocuvir Opticops (FDC)

Idoxuridine-

Ridinox (Bell Pharma), Toxil (Andre)

(ii) Ocular Anti-inflammatory-Antiallergics-

Sodium Cromoglycate-

Allercom (FDC), Allergo (Mejda), Cromol (Cipla), Fintal (Rallis), Ifiral (Unique)

Flurbiprofen-

Ocuflur (FDC), Cadiflur (Cadila Ph.), Flubinex (Torrent)

Betamethasone-

Betnesol E/E (Glaxo)

Tetrahydrozoline-

Visine (Pfizer)

Combinations-

Belmycetine-C (Bell), Betnor (Indoco), Betnesol-N (Glaxo), Chloramsone (Ranbaxy), Chlorocol-D (Jawa), Cortola-M (East-India), Cyclodex (Jawa), Dexona E/E (Cadila H.C.), Garasone (Fulford), Genticyn-B and H.C. (Nicholas), Pyricort, Pyrimon (FDC), Sofracort (Roussel).

(iii) Drugs for Glaucoma- Glaucoma is treated by the application of eye drops containing miotics, beta-blockers and by mouth with carbonic anhydrase inhibitors.

Pilocarpine-

Capromiotic (Bell), Pilocar (FDC), Andrecarpine (Andre)

Timolol-

Glaucare (Mejda), Iotim (FDC), Ocobar (PCI), Timolo (Bell)

Betaxolol-

Iobet (FDC), Optipres (Cipla), Nopres (Ochoa)

Acetazolamide-

Tab. Diamox (Wyeth), Actamide (Micro)

(iv) Mydriatics and Cyclopegics- These preparations dialates the pupil and paralyse the ciliary muscles.

Atropine-

Bellpinoatrin (Bell), Atropine (Jawa)

Homatropine-

Bell Homatropine (Bell), Homide (Warren)

Cyclopentolate-

Cyclomid (Jawa), Cyclogic (Mejda), Cyclogyl (Andre)

Tropicamide-

Tropicacyl (Sunways), Tropifrin (Jawa), Tropisyn (Mejda)

(v) Diagnostic and misc. Preparations-

New eye lotion (Optrex), Catalin (Glaxo), Cato-Bell, Tivision (Bell), Andre eye drops (Andre), Caracsol (Dey's), Drosyn (FDC), Profenac (Cipla), Oculose (Mejda), Zincula (Juggat),

(3) Ear

Drops and Ointments-

Otek, Otek-Ac, Otek-P (FDC), Otogesic (Ethnor), Tytin (Merind), Betnor Ear (Indoco), Genticyn, Genticyn-B, Genticyn-HC (Nicholas), Dexona (Cadila H.C.), Sofracort (Roussel), Chloromycetin (Parke-Davis), Methazil, Otoflour, Waxolve (Bell), Enteromycetin Otic (Dey's), Garamycin E/E (Fulford), Candid Ear (Glenmark), Paraxin Ear (Knoll)

(4) Nose and Oropharyngeal-

(i) Decongestants (With Antihistamines, Sympathomimetics)-

Oral-

Actifed (Wellcome), Cinaryl (Themis Pharma), Triminic (Wander), Contac-CC, Eskold (SB), Dristan (Wyeth), Cozy Plus (Ind-Swift),

Drops-

Dristan (Wyeth), Fenox (Knoll), Endrine (Wyeth), Fintal (Rallis).

(ii) Local Nasal Preparations-

Otrivin (Novartis), Nasivion (Merck), Decon (Cadila Ph.), Betnesol-N (Glaxo), Rhinocort (Astra-IDL)

(iii) Mouth Washes and Gum paints-

Betadine (Win-Medicare), Wokadine (Wockhardt), Dettolin (RCI), Alphadine (Nicholas), Steradent (RCI), Zytee (Reptakos), Kamillosan-N (German Remedies), Tantum Oral rinse (Elder), Stolin (Group) Mycoban (Pearch), Listerin (Parke-Davis)

(iv) Medicated Toothpastes-

Co-Q-Dent (Lupin), Senquel (Group), Senolin (Warren), Thermoseal (IPCA), Desent (Indoco), Toss (Ind-Swift), Emoform (J.L.Morison)

Section- B

CHAPTER- 12

Pharmacology

"Pharmacology" means the study of interactions between drugs and living cells. One aspect of pharmacology is concerned with the effects of drugs on body (cells, tissues, organs & system) is known as "Pharmacodynamics", where as the other aspects is concerned with the way drugs are handled by the body is known as "Pharmacokinetics".

"Toxicology" deals with the harmful & unwanted effects of drugs & "Therapeutics" deals with the study of drugs in men in disease conditons. The "Chemotherapy" is a special branch of therapeutics in which drugs are used to get rid of cancer cells or parasites.

Drugs sources are plants, animals, micro-organisms, minerals, human beings, and synthetic chemist's laboratory.

Drug

A drug is a substance used for the diagnosis, prevention, treatment or alleviation of the symptoms of disease.

Dose

The dose of a drug is a quantity necessary to produce certain measaurable bio-chemical or physiological changes in the body.

It is expressed in terms of:

(i) Weight (gm.,mg.,mcg.)

(ii) Volume (ml.)

(iii) Satandard units

Therapeutic Index

The therapeutic index refers to the relative margin of safety a drug possesses.

Teratogenic Drugs

The drugs that reach the developing embryo and foetus during the early period of pregnancy when organs are being formed, can cause congenital defects.

Dosage Forms

For administration, drugs are made into "Formulations" or "Dosage Forms" that are stable, acceptable and effective. Below written are improtant dosage forms

(i) Tablets- They can be of various shapes & sizes (viz. round, oval, caplet) and may be plain, sugar coated, film coated or enteric coated. The enteric coating may be employed for drugs which irritate the stomach or are destroyed by the gastric secretions. To make a drug into a tablet form the inert substances are mixed with them, called "excipients".

(ii) Capsules- They are soft or hard shells of gelatin containing active drugs. The excipients used in capsules, are called "fillers".

(iii) Injections- They are sterile solutions, or suspensions, or powder (to be dissolved or suspended in a suitable vehicle). These fluid preparations are meant for administration either I.V. (Intravenous) or I.M. (Intra muscular) or subcutaneous, etc., through a hollow needle.

(iv) Mixtures- The mixtures are liquid medications to be taken by mouth. Physically a mixture may be a solution, a suspension or an emulsion.

The sweet mixtures are called "syrups", where as those contain alcohol are called "elixirs".

(v) Lozenges- These are tablets intended for sucking and generally contain anaesthetic or antiseptic drugs for local effect in the mouth and throat.

(vi) Creams & Ointments- These are semisolid, pasty preparations in which the active drug is dissolved or dispersed. The water-miscible base preparation, called 'creams' and greasy base preparation, called 'ointments'.

(vii) Lotions- They are aqueous solutions or suspensions meant for local application.

(viii) Liniments- They have an oily, alcoholic or hydroalcoholic base preparation also meant for local application.

(ix) Drops- They are liquid solutions or suspensions meant for oral use or for local use in eye, ear or nose.

(x) Powders- The active drug is diluted in inert substance such as starch or lactose and meant for oral use or for local application.

(xi) Inhalers- These formulations yield a fine mist of particles or droplets for inhalation.

(xii) Suppositories- They are bullet shaped, solid dosage forms meant for insertion into the vagina or the rectum and provide local action.

(xiii) Enemas- These are fluid preparation given rectally, either for washing out the colon (evacuation enemas), or for local action in the colon (retention enemas). Sometimes glcouse and salt solutions are given rectally for absorption.

The drugs can be applied, used or administered in a numbers of ways depending upon the situations, viz. oral route, sublingual route (placed under the tongue), injections (I.V., I.M., subcutaneous, intra-articular, intrapleural, intrathaceal, intraperitoneal), local application, inhalation & rectal route. Rarely, drugs are injected into arteries (intra-arterial).

Posology

The study of determining dose is known as "Posology". The amount of drug administered at one time is known as "dose". The size and frequency of dose depends upon age , body weight, route of administration, severity of disease and individual's tolerance, hyper- sensitivity & intolerance.

Bioavailability

It is the actual quantity of the drug available for action in the body or the blood stream. Genrally, the bioavailability for a solid formulation is proportional to its dissolution rate, which in turn is governed by a variety of chemical, physical and pharmaceutical factors.

Drug Distribution

The diffusion of the drug from the blood stream to the other compartments (tissues/organs) of the body, through extracellular fluid or both extra and intracellular fluid.

Drug Transfer

The transfer of drug from various compartments of the body to the excretory compartments.

Half-Life

The half life or biological half life of a drug means the time during which half the administered dose (50%) is eliminatied from the body. Slower the rate of elimination of a drug, longer will be its half life.

Plasma Half Life

The interval during which the plasma level of a drug falls to half of its original value.

Pharmacodynamics

It is the experimental study of drug effects on the living cells, and it deals with the interaction between the chemical components of the living systems and the drugs, including their mechanism of action.

Pharmacokinetics

It is concerned with the way drugs are handled by the body viz. absorption, distribution and elimination of the drugs.

(i) Absorption of drugs- The absorption of the drugs into the blood occurs through the epithelial surfaces and capillary walls (except for injected drugs through a vein or an artery). The drug firstly dissolve in the fluid covering the epithelia or the tissue fluid surrouding the capillaries. The dissolution rate depends upon the size of drug particle (e.g. micronised drugs are absorbed more rapidly & completely).

(ii) Distribution of drugs- After absorption of the drug into the blood, it spread to the tissues or organs of the body. Substances which have very large molecules and can't easily pass through capillary walls remain confined to the blood. And if a drug gets bound to plasma proteins (mainly albumin), the bound fraction also remains in the blood until it gets free again.

Some drugs cannot enter cells easily and so they spread through the extracellular fluid only. However many drugs spread through out the body water and enter cells.

Some drugs pass across cerebrospinal fluid, the brain and the foetal circulation easily, some with difficulty and some not at all. Some drugs are selectively concentrated in specific tissues or organs only.

(iii) Elimination of drugs- The most important pathway of drug elimination is excretion through the kidneys, either by glomerular filtration or by tubular secretion.

The elimination of the drugs, other than the kidneys, may be through skin, lungs, G.I. tract (faeces), bile and during lactation through milk.

Drugs Metabolism

Some drugs are excerted unchanged, however, many drugs undergo some chemical changes before excretion. Liver is the principal organ where drugs are metabolised and the enzymes in the liver cells which catalyze the biotransformation of drugs are known as "microsomal enzymes". Other tissues which can metabolize drugs are the plasma, the kidneys and the gastrointestinal epithelium.

Some drugs, which become active after a metabolic alteration in the body, are called "pro drugs", where as in most cases the chemical changes result in the formation of compounds that are inactive or less active, less lipid soluble and easy to eliminate.

The factors influencing the drug metabolism are diseases of the liver, severe malnutrition, old age, in premature babies, & genetic variation and requires lower than usual dose.

Some drugs are capable of including the formation of drug metabolizing enzymes in the liver and enhance not only their own metabolism but also that of other drugs given with them.

Some drugs are oxidised to form oxides, hydroxides, sulphoxides, etc. Some drugs are reduced by the addition of hydrogen or hydrolyzed or combined with other substances.

Drug Interaction

When two or more drugs are given concomitantly, they may influence each other with respect to absorption, distribution, metabolism, elimination and the concentration at the site of action , so that drug effect may be diminished, shortened, enhanced or prolonged.

Drug Action

The action means the basic or primary changes which occur at the level of cells or molecules in the protoplasm.

Majority of the drugs have a systemic action (except drugs have a local action) and being absorbed into the blood & carried to their target organ or tissue. Drugs either "stimulate" cells (an increase in the physiological function of the cell) or "inhibit" cells (a decrease in the physiological function of the cell), they cannot impart any new function on the cell.

The action of the drug may be 'simple physical phenomenon' or a 'chemical action'. But most of the drugs exerts a 'biological action'. In biological action the drug brings about complex physico -chemical changes in the molecules of cell membrane & protoplasm. The molecules which serve as the point of contact for a drug in the target cells are called,"receptors" and the drugs which make contact with receptors are called "agonists". Some drugs merely occupy the receptors and prevent agonists from doing their job are called, "antagonists or blockers".

Drug Effects

The effects means the secondary changes which results from the action, for example the action of an antibiotic is to impair some vital metabolic process in the bacterial cell, the effect may vary from slowing of growth, complete inhibition of growth or even to the cell's death.

The combined drug effect of two drugs may be equal to the sum of their individual effects (addition), greater than the sum (potentiation), or less than the sum (antagonism) or complementary in a therapeutic sense (synergism).

(i) Addition- When two drugs brings about the same effect through the same action.

(ii) Potentiation- When two drugs brings about the greater than the sum of their individual effects through different actions.

(iii) Antagonism- The reduction of the effect of one drug (agonist) by another drug (antagonist).

(iv) Synergism- The effect of two drugs is complementary in a therapeutic sense.

Drug Tolerance and Resistance

When more and more of a drug is needed to produce the same effect , the phenomenon is called "tolerance".

The tolerance of micro-organisms to antibiotics and chemotherapeutic agents is called "resistance".

Unwanted Effects of Drug

'Side effects' means those known unwanted pharmacological effects of a drug in usual doses. This term is some times used loosely to mean any unwanted effect that is mild (and) annoying but not harmful. When an unwanted effect is severe in intensity and potentially harmful; it is usually described as a 'toxic effect'. A comprehensive and widely used term which covers all unwanted drug effect is called "adverse drug reaction".

The adverse drug reaction can be due to hypersensitivity, over dosage, intolerance, organ toxicity, teratogenicity, superinfection, photosensitization, etc.

Prescription Terms

The commonly used terms by the doctors while prescribing drugs are listed below:

I.M.	=	Intramuscularly
I.V.	=	Intravenously
S.C.	=	Subcutaneously
P.O. (Per orum)	=	Orally, by mouth
O.D.(omni die)	=	Once a day
B.D. (bis die)	=	Twice a day
T.I.D. (ter in die)	=	Three times a day
Q.I.D.(quater in die)	=	Four times a day
H.S.(hora somni)	=	At bed time
a.c.(anti cibum)	=	Before food
p.c. (post cibum)	=	After food
S.O.S.(si opus sit)	=	When needed
Stat. (statim)	=	Immediately, at once
ad. lib. (ad libitum)	=	As much as desired
p.r.n. (pro re nata)	=	As occasion requires
Mist. (mistura)	=	Mixture
Gutta (guttae)	=	Drops
Q.S. (quantum sufficiat)	=	Sufficient quantity
dil (dilutus)	=	Dilute
ung. (unguentum)	=	Ointment

Section- B

CHAPTER- 13

Microbiology

Microbiology is the study of "microbes", or microscopic living organisms. Almost all the micro-organisms are smaller than 0.1 mm. in diameter. The microbes of medical interest include "Protozoa" (Amoeba-the smallest organism), "Fungi" (including moulds and yeasts), "Bacteria" and "Viruses".

Only a small proportion of the micro-organisms that abound in nature are disease producing for human being. Majority of micro-organisms feed on dead organic matter and are termed as "Saprophytes" and other can survive only in the company of living cells, either on them or inside them and are termed as "Parasites".

A parasite is defined as micro-organism or larger species (e.g.round worms, thread worms, hook worms, guinea worms, etc.), that lives in or on another animal and obtains its nourishment from a living host.

Parasitic micro-organisms are either commensals (harmless) or pathogens (harmful). The commensals constitute the normal flora of the healthy body. They live on the skin and on the mucus membranes of the upper respiratory tract, the intestines and the vagina. They are generally harmless and preventing the growth of disease-producing micro-organisms; in addition, some commensals in the gut produce vitamins. But under certain circumstances, the commensals may invade the tissues and cause disease, thus acting as opportunistic pathogens.

True pathogens are the parasitic micro-organisms which invade tissues and cause disease. The process of microbial invasion of the body is called "Infection", disease is often called as "Infective Disease". Those infective diseases that are readily communicable from person to person by direct or indirect contact are called "Infectious or Contagious Disease".

In general, micro-organisms require a source of carbohydrate to provide energy, a source of nitrogen and various minerals & vitamins to regulate metabolic reactions. Some bacteria need substances which are essential for their life process but which they are unable to synthesise, are called "Essential Growth Factors".

Carrier of Micro-Organism

Following are the carrier of micro-organism:

(i) Human beings (ii) Animals (iii) Water
(iv) Food (v) Air (vi) Dust, etc.

Broad Classfication of Micro-Organism

The micro-organism can be classified as:

(i) Protozoa (Entamoeba histolytica)

(ii) Fungus

(iii) Schizomycetes (Rickettsiae, Viruses, Bacteria, Mycoplasma, Chlamydiae)

(i) Protozoa- The word protozoon (singular) means the first animal. An amoeba is the simplest and most common of all protozoa. The protozoa size ranges from 2 to 200 microns.

Some forms of protozoa

(a) Amoeba (b) Giardia (c) Trypanosoma
(d) Leishmania (e) Trichomonas (f) Balantidium coli, etc.

Several protozoa cause diseases in human & other animals. Some amoeba live inside our intestines and are harmless, whereas some cause diseases e.g. dysentery. Protozoa donot posses a cell wall. They are found in moist habitats viz.- sea, soil, fresh water. However, for the sake of convenience some forms of protozoa will be described at the end of this chapter.

(ii) Fungus- The fungi are both unicellular and multicellular. They can form spores and generally reproduce both sexually as well as asexually by binnary fission, budding and regeneration from fragments.

Some very important medicines such as Penicillin are made from the fungi, where as some fungi cause diseases like candidiasis, athlet's foot and ring worm.

Fungi consist of two main groups of organisms:

(a) Yeast- They are usually unicellular, range in size from 5 to 10 microns. They can survive in both aerobic and anaerobic conditions.

(b) Moulds- They are multicellular and have a filament like appearance, e.g. mushrooms. They can survive in aerobic conditions.

(iii) Schizomycetes- A group of micro-organisms , called schizomycetes. These includes

(a) Viruses- They are the smallest living organisms & can be described as tiny envelops of nucleic acid, either D.N.A.(Small pox, Chicken pox, Herpes simplex, Herpes Zoster) or R.N.A.(Poliomyelitis, Mumps, Measels, Rabies), but never both. Viruses can not be seen by simple microscopes because their size ranges from 0.015 to 0.2 micron. They donot grow on their own, but can only multiply inside another host organism such as bacteria, plants or animal cells.

Viruses are not like other micro-organisms which possess a cell body & other structures. Indeed, their very name is derived from the respective host or from the disease that they cause, e.g. measle virus cause measles in humans, viral dysentary, chicken pox virus, influenza virus, mumps virus, etc. It is believed that some cancers are also caused by viruses.

Common cold, flu (Influenza) or viral fever, rabies are the common diseases of viruses.

(b) Rickettsiae- These are unicellular micro-organsims, in size they are larger than viruses but smaller than bacteria. They grow only inside the living cells. Rockey mountain fever, Q-fever are the common disease of Rickettsiae, which are found very rare in India.

(c) Mycoplasma- They assume various forms as they lack in a rigid cell wall and very exacting nutritional requirements are the characteristics of these organisms. An example is Mycoplasma pneumoniae.

(d) Chlamydiae- These organisms differ from viruses, as they contain both types of nucleic acid (D.N.A. & R.N.A.). They are also known as Bedsoniae. An example is Chalamydia trachomatis.

(e) Bacteria- These are uni-cellular micro-organisms, in size about 1 micron in transverse diameter. They have a rigid cell wall, protoplasm but no well-defined nucleus. They reproduce by a

sexual method known as binary fission. Examples are Staphylococcus aureus, Enterococci, Salmonella typhi, E-coli, etc.

Structure of Bacteria

The bacterium has a "Cell Membrane", out side the cell membrane, there is a rigid "Cell Wall". The cell wall is absent in Viruses, Rickettsiae, Mycoplasma and L-forms Bacteria. The bacterial cells have a homogeneous, colourless protoplasm bounded by a cell membrane. There is no distinct nucleus, the genetic chromatin material being dispersed throughout the protoplasm.

Types of Bacteria

Certain bacteria are capable of free movements. They owe their motility to hair-like processes, known as "Flagella", which arise in the protoplasm and pass out through the cell-wall.

In some bacteria there are small hair-like structures surrounding the cell wall, known as "Pilated bacteria".

Some bacteria have a layer of jelly-like substance surrounding the cell wall, known as "Capsulated bacteria".

Environment for Bacteria

The bacterial growth requires:

(i) O_2 and/or CO_2 concentration

(ii) Enzymes

(iii) pH concentration

(iv) Temperature

(v) Moisture

At different enviornment in the host, the commensal bacteria become opportunistic pathogens.

Nomenclature and Classification of Bacteria

There are so many different types of bacteria with so many different types of Latin names that it would be difficult to remember all of them after one or many readings.

Bacteria are named according to their shapes, arrangement in which they lie on a slide, correspond to the organs from which they come, etc.

The names of micro-organisms consist of two words, e.g. "Treponema pallidum". The first word indicates the genus & its first letter is written as a captial; the second word stand for the species & its first letter is written in small letter.

Within each species of micro-organisms there are clans or strains which differ from one another in their susceptibility to various antibiotics and the type of antibody they induce.

Bacteria are classified according to their:

(a) Staining characteristics

(b) Shape & arrangement

(c) Growth requirement

(d) Genetic characteristics

(a) Staining Characteristics

The stain usually used is called "Gram's stain", which is a mixture of two stains. The smear is treated first with methyl violet followed by iodine. It is then decolourised with alcohol and washed with water. Finally it is counterstained with carbol fuchsin.

Bacteria which take up & retain the first violet stain are called "Gram-positive", those which take up the red counterstain are called "Gram-negative".

The other type of stain is called "Ziehl-Neelsen stain". This is employed to identify the "acid-fast" organisms (e.g. Mycobacterium tuberculosis, M. leprae). The smear is first treated with hot carbol fuchsin & then decolourized with sulphuric acid. Finally methylene blue is added and the excess washed away with water. The bacteria which retain the first red stain inspite of acid treatment, are called "Acid-Fast Bacteria".

(b) Shape & Arrangement

A spherical bacterium is called "Coccus" (Micrococci) & if pairs are formed called "Diplococci". While multiplying, a coccus may form a bunch like that of grapes, called "Staphylococci". If it forms a chain, called "Streptococci".

A rod-shaped bacterium is called "Bacillus" and a oval - shaped bacterium is called "Cocco-bacilli". The comma-shaped is called "Vibro". The Spirochaete is spiral in shape.

(c) Growth Requirement

Some bacteria require O_2 to live and are called "Aerobes "(e.g. Staphylococci). Some can live in less O_2 & are called "Anaerobes" (e.g. C. tetani). Some can live both in the presence or absence of O_2 and are called "Facultative anaerobes (e.g. E-coli).

Some can live only in the absence of O_2 and are called "Obligate anaerobes" (e.g. Bacteroides fragilis), where as some require CO_2 to live & are called "Capnophillic" (e.g. N. meningitidis).

(d) Genetic Characteristics

All the bacteria belong to a kingdom called Procaryote, further having family, genus & species e.g.

Pseudomonaciae	=	Family
Pseudomonas	=	Genus
Aeruginosa	=	Species

Beta-Lactamase Enzymes

Shortly after the introduction of Penicillin, resistance among Staphylococcus aureus was noted. Such resistance is due to enzymatic inactivation of the beta-lactam ring of the Penicillin molecule. The responsible enzyme is known as "Pencillinase", although it is only one of an ever increasing number of enzymes identified and collectively known as "Beta-Lactamases".

The beta-lactamases are widely distributed among Gram-negative bacteria and varies among different bacteria.

Infection

It is the successful invasion, establishment and growth of micro-organisms in the tissue of the host.

Sources of Infection

The sources of infection are the habitats in which the pathogenic microbes ordinarily grow and from which they are disseminated to susceptible hosts. The objects which carry pathogens in a surviving, but non-growing conditions, are known as "Vehicles" of infection. Many species of pathogens are derived mainly from ill patients as their source, but many others grow in and are disseminated from healthy persons, known as "Carriers", in whom they cause only a limited clinical infection (e.g. Amoebiasis, Typhoid fever).

Process of Infection

(i) Inoculation- The transfer or an introduction of the living virus or bacteria into the tissue. For example the transfer of bacteria to respiratory tract and then to other parts of the body.

(ii) Incubation- The stage in which bacteria multiply in the body without the appearance of symptoms of disease.

(iii) Acute Phase- Suddenly short and severe symptoms of disease start and the beginning stage is called acute phase.

(iv) Convalescence- The host defence mechanism over come and eliminate pathogens from the tissue and the host recovers.

(v) Chronic Phase- The stage in which sign and symptoms of the infection are continuing for a long time.

Normal Sign and Symptoms of Infection

(i) Chills (Unpleasant cold feeling)

(ii) Malaise (A feeling of illness and discomfort)

(iii) Headache

(iv) Aching muscles

(v) Elevated W.B.C. count

(vi) Elevated heart rate

Types of Infection

(i) Primary Infection (Ist Infection caused by one pathogen)

(ii) Secondary or super Infection (Ist Infection is added by another infection)

(iii) Mixed Infection (Caused by 2 or more pathogens)

(iv) Opportunity Infection (Caused by commensals)

(v) Nosocomial Infection (Caused when a patient has been in hospital for atleast 72 hours and did not have signs & symptoms of such infection on admission)

(vi) Recurrent Infection (Occurs repeatedly due to abnormal organ structure)

(vii) Re-infection (After recovery, caused by different pathogen)

(viii) Community Acquired Infection (Caused by other than hospital environment)

Pathogenicity

It means the capacity to produce disease or pathology. The mere infection (invasion of pathogen into the body), does not mean that disease will follow. For disease to develop, either the host body defence must be subdued or the pathogen must possess a high digree of ability to overcome host defence, invade tissues, produces lesions and disturb function (Virulence).

There are two properties which constitute virulence are "Invasiveness" and "Toxigenicity".

Invasiveness means the capacity to spread through tissues. To a large extent it is due to the production of enzymes (e.g. Coagulase by Staphylococci, Streptokinase by Streptococci, etc.) by pathogens which break down the ground substance in tissues.

The toxins produced by bacteria are "Exotoxins" and "Endotoxins". The exotoxins are powerful poisons, released by living micro-organism in the surrounding medium. They are susceptible to distruction by heat, are strongly antigenic and can be treated with formalin to form "Toxoids" (Protective vaccines that are antigenic but nontoxic e.g. Diphtheria and Tetanus toxoids).

Endotoxins are those that escape from the bacterial cell when it dies and disintegrates and are comparatively less potent poisons and cannot be made into toxoids. They are released by many gram negative bacteria.

Body Response to Infection

The body's reaction to infection is seen not only at the site of Infection but often in the whole body.

In the Infected tissue the pathogen and its products act as irritants and set up inflammation. It may be acute as in Pneumonia or chronic as in Tuberculosis.

It also sets up fever (caused due to the action of bacterial toxins and products of tissue necrosis, on the brains heat regulating centre), rise in W.B.C. count (Leucocytosis) and production of antibodies, all of which help the body to dispose of the invading pathogens.

Antimicrobials

The substances which can be given from outside, to help the body to fight the infection. For more detail see chapter 14 of Section-B.

Nomenclature of Infection

Infections are usually named according to the organ which has been infected. For example few infections are listed below:

(a) Brain (Encephalos)	-	Encephalitis
(b) Covering of brain (Meninges)	-	Meningitis
(c) Tongue (Glosso)	-	Glossitis
(d) Throat (Pharynx)	-	Pharyngitis
(e) Larynx	-	Laryngitis

(f) Sinus	-	Sinusitis
(g) Ear	-	Otitis
(h) Lung (Pneumo)	-	Pneumonitis or Pneumonia
(i) Covering of lungs (Pleura)	-	Pleuritis
(j) Breathing tube (Bronchus)	-	Bronchitis
(k) Stomach (Gastro)	-	Gastritis
(l) Intestines (Entero)	-	Enteritis
(m) Lower bowel (Colon)	-	Colitis
(n) Appendix	-	Appendicitis
(o) Liver (Hepatic)	-	Hepatitis
(p) Heart muscle (Myocardium)	-	Myocarditis
(q) Muscle (Myo)	-	Myositis
(r) Skin (Derma)	-	Dermatitis, and so on

This is only a small list, but the general principle seems to be to add an "itis" after the concerned organ.

The nomenclature of infections is based on the name of the organ and does not indicate the pathogens responsible for the infection, as this is not always possible.

Common Parasitic Diseases

The disease caused by the pathogenic parasite is called "parasitic disease". The common parasites are:

(1) Protozoa- Unicellular organisms

(2) Metazoa- Multicellular organisms (Helminth)

(1) Common Protozoal Diseases

(a) Intestinal protozoal diseases e.g. -Amoebiasis, Giardiasis, Trichomoniasis, Balantidiasis.

(b) Systemic protozoal diseases e.g. Malaria, Kala-Azar (Visceral Leishmaniasis), Trypanosomiasis.

(i) Malaria

Malaria is a parasitic disease caused by the protozoan of the genus "Plasmodium" which is transmitted into man by the female "Anopheles mosquito".

The World over, malaria is the most common cause of morbidity and mortality from infection in man.

Types of malaria

(a) Malignant tertian (MT) malaria- is caused by Plasmodium falciparum.

(b) Benign tertian (BT) malaria- is caused by Plasmodium vivax.

(c) Quartan (Q) malaria- is caused by Plasmodium malariae.

(d) Ovale tertian (OT) malaria- is caused by Plasmodium ovale.

The term tertian indicates that the atack of chills and fever typically tend to recur every third day. The infection caused by P. vivax, P. malariae and P. ovale are classified as "Relapsing malarias" because they have a secondary exoerythrocytic stage of development which provides a reservoir of parasites for the reinfection of erythrocytes. In contrast P. flaciparum has no exoerythrocytic stage in its life cycle.

Life cycle of Plasmodium (In human)

The plasmodium runs its asexual cycle in man (causing pathogenic effect) and the sexual cycle in the mosquito. The human phase begins when an infected female Anopheles mosquito bites man & injects "sporozoites" from her salivary glands. The injected sporozoites rapidly leave the circulation and localize in the liver parenchyma cells and develop into "Primary tissue schizonts". The primary tissue schizonts mature with-in 8-21 days & form "Merozoites", at this stage the subject remains symptom free.

On maturity, the merozoites liberate from liver cells & invade the erythrocytes. At the end of erythrocytic cycle the infected red blood cells rupture, releasing merozoites, pigments and other products into the blood. This point of time marks the clinical attack of malaria mainfested by chills, fever and profound sweating.

After several cycles some erythrocytic parasites differentiate into male & female "Gametocytes", that may be ingested by a female Anopheles mosquito from the blood stream of the infected individual, to start its sexual cycle in the gut of mosquito. Hence the cycle is completed.

(ii) Kala-Azar

Kala-Azar or Visceral Leishmaniasis is caused by the protozoal parasite called the Leishmania donovani. This is transmitted into man from the cattle or a diseased person by a bloodsucking sandfly. Treatment involves drugs such as, Stibamine glucoside or Ethylstibamine, or Sodium antimony gluconate, or Hydroxystilbamidine isethionate, or Pentamidine isethionate are used.

(iii) Trypanosomiasis

It is a term applied to disease caused by the protozoa of the genus "Trypanosoma". Aferican sleeping sickness is caused by T. gambiense and T. rhodesiense. South American sleeping sickness is caused by T. cruzii. It is transmitted by the blood sucking tsetse fly. If untreated may lead to the manifestation of meningoencephalitis. Treated by drugs such as, Melarsoprol (Mel B), or Melarsonyl (Mel W), or Suramin, or Pentamidine, or Propamidine .

(iv) Giardiasis

Giardiasis (Lambliasis) is caused by "Giardia lamblia', a protozoan which may occur in the gastrointestinal tract. Treatment involved drugs such as Metronidazole, or Tinidazole, or Chloroquine, or Diiodohydroxyquin, and Hydroxychloroquine are used.

(v) Balantidiasis

Balantidiasis or Ciliate dysentery is caused by "Balantidium coli". Treatment involved drugs such as Tetracyclines, or Oxytetracycline, or Diiodohydroxyquin and Emetine are used.

(vi) Trichomoniasis

It is caused by the protozoa of the genus "Trichomona". Trichomona intestinalis enters in the human body along with contaminated food or drink; where as T. vaginalis causes white vaginal discharge (sexually transmitted in the female). Ideal specific drugs are Metronidazole or Tinidazole orally which should be taken simultaneously by both the marital partners. Topical preparations such as Silver nitrate or Furazolidine are also used generally.

(vii) Amoebiasis

Amoebiasis is an infection caused by "Entamoeba histolytica". There are two principal form in which it can exist, viz.-"Trophozoites" and "Cyst".

Trophozoites are the active, motile, vegetative form which move about by extending finger like projections called "pseudopodia".The trophozoites are ineffective in transmitting infection, as they are easily distroyed by heat, gastric acid and do not survive long outside the host.

In the host G.I. tract, some trophozoites secrete a tough wall around them and form cyst. The cyst can live for long periods, both outside the body and within the human intestine. They are capable of transmitting infection to a new host. The cyst are also resistant to gastric acid.

Life cycle-

The disease is transmitted when mature cysts are ingested. On entering the small intestine, the cysts lose their thick wall in the alkaline environment and each cyst develops into 8 trophozoites, usually in the ileocaecal region of the intestine. This process takes about 4-5 day's.

The trophozoite invade the intestinal mucosa causing ulceration (amoebic dysentery), diarrhoea and abdominal pain. The trophozoites release a substance that digests mucosal cells and finally they may find their way to the mesenteric veins to be carried to the liver by the portal circulation & causing amoebic hepatitis and liver abscess. Rarely, the trophozoites may spread through blood stream to distant organs such as the brain. Thus, the trophozoite form is responsible for both the intestinal and extra-intestinal symptoms of amoebiasis.

Some of the trophozoites present in the lumen of the colon secrete a wall around them & become cysts. In due course these cysts are passed out in the faeces, infect a new host and propagate the species by starting a new life cycle.

Amoebiasis in man presents as:

(a) Asymptomatic intestinal infection

(b) Mild to moderate intestinal infection

(c) Severe intestinal infection (dysentery)

(d) Amoebic liver abscess

(e) Amoeboma or extraintestinal infection (amoebic brain abscess, amoebic lung abscess).

(2) Common Metazoal Diseases

The helminths (multicellular organsims) infecting man belong to varied zoological species, with marked differences in their body structure, physiology, habitat in the human host and sensitivity to drugs. In man they are located in the intestinal tract or other tissues.

There are three categories of worms, namely "Nematodes", "Cestodes" and "Trematodes" parasitize man. Infection with more than one type of worm is common.

Nematodes- The nematodes are:

Ascaris lumbricoides (round worm)

Enterobius vermicularis (pin worm)

Trichuris trichuria (whip worm)

Strongyloides stercoralis (thread worm)

Ancylostoma duodenale & Necator americans (hook worm)

Wuchereria bancrofti, W. malayi (filarial worms)

Dracunculus medinensis (guinea worm).

Cestodes- The cestodes are:

Taenia saginata (beef tape worm)

Taenia solium (pork tape worm)

Hymenolepis nana (dwarf tape worm)

Diphyllobothrium latum (fish tape worm)

Trematodes-The common trematodes are:

Liver flukes, Lung flukes, Intestinal flukes, Blood flukes.

The anthelmintics used (Vermicide or Vermifuge) against the intestinal helminths, kill or sterilize the worms or paralyse them so that they lose hold of the intestinal mucosa and are expelled via the faeces.

Table - 4 Important Human Pathogens

Group	Micro- organism	Disease
Protozoa	Plasmodium	Malaria
	Giardia lamblia	Giardiasis
	Trichomonas vaginalis	Trichomoniasis
	Entamoeba histolytica	Amoebiasis, Dysentery, Liver abscess.
Fungi	Candida albicans	Candidiasis of the skin and mucous membranes (e.g. Vaginitis)
	Dermatophytes (e.g. Trichophyton, Epidermophyton)	Tinea infection (Ring worm) of skin, hair and nails.

	Aspergillus niger	Bronchopneumonia, Lung abscess
	Histoplasma capsulatum	Histoplasmosis, involving lungs and viscera.
	Cryptococcus neoformans	Cryptococcosis, involving CNS.
Viruses	DNA viruses (e.g. Chicken pox virus, Herpes simplex virus, etc.)	Small pox, Chickenpox, Genital Herpes, Herpeszoster, Keratoconjunctivitis.
	RNA viruses (e.g. Influenza virus A, Mumps virus)	Common Cold, Influenza, Mumps, Dengue fever, Gastroenteritis, Rabies, Poliomyelitis, Meningitis.
	Unidentified viruses	Infective hepatitis, Serum hepatitis.
Rickettsiae	Rickettsia	Typhus fever, Q. fever, Rocky mountain-spotted fever.
Mycoplasma	Mycoplasma pneumoniae	Bronchitis, Pneumonia.
	Mycoplama hominis	Nonspecific urethritis/ vaginitis.
Unclassified	Chlamydia psittaci	Psittacosis
	Chlamydia trachomatis	Trachoma, Inclusion conjuctivitis, Nonspecific urethritis, Lymphogranuloma - venereum.
Bacteria	(i) Gram-positive cocci :	
	Staphylococcus aureus Staphylococcus albus	Abscesses, Bacteraemia, Boils, Osteomyelitis, Cellulitis, Pneumo nia, Meningitis, Endocarditis.
	Pneumococcus	Pneumonia, Otitis, Meningitis
	Streptococcus pyogenes	Impetigo, Cellulitis, U.R.T.I, L.R.T.I. Gynaec infections.
	Streptococcus viridans	Dental abscess, Endocarditis, U.T.I.
	Streptococcus faecalis	Wound infections, U.T.I. Endocarditis.
	(ii) Gram-positive bacilli :	
	Bacillus anthracis (Anthrax)	Malignant postule, Pneumonia, Meningitis.
	Corynebacterium diptheriae	Diptheria.
	Clostridium tetani	Tetanus
	Clostridium welchii/ septicum	Gas gangrene.
	Listeria monocytogenes	Recurrent abortion, Bacteraemia, Meningitis
	(iii) Gram - negative cocci:	
	Neisseria genorrhoeae	Gonorrhoea
	Neisseria meningitidis	Meningitis, Bacteraemia.
	(iv) Gram- negative bacilli:	
	Escherichia coli (E-coli)	U.T.I., Gastroenteritis, Bacteraemia.
	Entoerobacter aerogenes	U.T.I., and other infections.

Bacteria Contd.	Klebsiella pneumoniae	Pneumonia.
	Klebsiella aerogenes	U.T.I.
	Proteus mirabilis/ vulgaris	U.T.I. and other infections.
	Haemophilius influnzae	R.T.I., Meningitis.
	Haemophilius ducreyi	Chancroid.
	Pseudomonas aeruginosa	U.T.I., Respiratory and Skin infec tions.
	Salmonella typhosa	Typhoid fever
	Other Salmonella species	Paratyphoid fever, Gastroenteritis.
	Shigella species	Bacillary dysentery
	Vibrio cholerae	Cholera.
	Spirillum minus	Rat-bite fever
	Bordetella pertusis	Whooping cough
	Pasturella pestis	Plague
	Bacteroides fragilis	Wound infections, Abscesses, Septicaemia.
	(v) Acid- Fact bacilli :	
	Mycobacterium tuberculosis	Tuberculosis (Pulmonary)
	Mycobacterium leprae	Leprosy
	(vi) Spirochetes :	
	Treponema pallidum	Syphilis
	Treponema pertenuae	Yaws
	Leptospira	Weil's disease
	Borrelia recurrentis	Relapsing fever
	Borrelia vincenti	Vincent's angina
	(vii) Actinomycetes :	
	Actinomyces israelii	Actinomycosis of jaws, lungs, intestines
	Nocardia asteroides	Nocardiosis
	Nocardia madurae	Madura foot

Clinical Aspects

Abscess- It is a localized collection of pus produced by pyogenic organisms. It may be acute or chronic.

Ascariasis- The infestation by the Ascarides. Affects bowel & may also spread to the stomach, liver & lungs.

Bacteraemia- The prescence of living bacteria in the blood.

Bilharziasis-The infection of the human body caused by blood flukes, infested from drinking, or bathing in infected water.

Chickenpox- A mild, specific infection caused by Varicella-zoster virus.

Commensal- A parasitic micro-organism adapted to grow on body surfaces of the host, forming part of the normal flora. Generally are harmless.

Dengue fever- The infection is caused by an arbovirus conveyed by a mosquito. It is characterized by fever, rheumatic pain & a skin eruption.

Dracontiasis- The infestation is caused by Dracunculus medinesis or Guinea worm, a nematode parasite which infests man from contaminated drinking water.

Filariasis- The infestation is caused by Wuchereria bancrofti, a nematode parasite which is transmitted by the culex mosquito.

Gas gangrene- It is mainly caused by anaerobic micro-organisms Clostridium welchii,in which a wound is infected , normally found in the intestine.

Herpes-The vasicular eruption caused due to a virus infection. Herpes simplex virus causes genital herpes, dendritic cornel ulcer & cold sores around the mouth. Herpes zoster virus attacks sensory nerves, with severe pain and appearance of vesicles along the distribution of the nerves involved.

Influenza- An acute viral infection of the nasopharynx & respiratory tract which occurs in epidemic or pandemic form.

Leprosy- A progressive & contagious disease caused by Mycobacterium leprae, characterized by granulomatous formation in the nerves or on the skin.

Madura foot- A disease of the foot characterized by the swelling and the development of nodules & sinuses.

Mumps- It is an acute specfic inflammation of the parotid glands, caused by a virus.

Poliomyelitis- It is an epidemic virus infection which attacks the motor neurones of the anterior horns in the brain stem and spinal cord. It also known as infantile paralysis.

Rabies- It is a fatal infection in man caused by a virus. The infection follows the bite of a rabid animal (Dog, Cat, Fox).

Smallpox- It is caused by a virus, now eradicated from the most parts of the world.

Tetanus- It is caused by Clostridium tatani, an anaerobic which may be present in road dust and manure. The patients develops spasm and rigidity of muscles.

Tuberculosis- It is a chronic infection caused by Mycobacterium tuberculosis and occasionally by M. bovis. Infection of the upper lung is the most common form of tuberculosis. Tuberculosis Meningitis, Pericarditis, Peritonitis and Osteomyelitis are the acute systemic non-pulmonary forms.

Typhoid fever- It is an infectious fever usually spread by contamination of food, milk or water supplies with Salmonella typhi, either directly by sewage, indirectly by flies or by faulty personal hygiene. Its average incubation period is 10 to 14 days.

Weil's disease- It is a type of jaundice with fever caused by Leptospira-icterohaemorrhagica.

Yaws- It is a tropical disease caused by Treponema pertenuae which resembles syphilis so closely that they may be one and the same disease.

Applied Medicines

(i) Anti fungal-

Griseofulvin-

Idifulvin (IDPL), Grisovin-FP (Glaxo), Fluvin (Bombay Tab.)

Nystatin-

Mycostatin Tab. (Sarabhai)

Fluconazole-

Fluzon (Lesante), Forcan (Cipla), Zocon (FDC), Fluzide (Concept), Antif (Twilight), Flutrox (Dabur), Syscan (Torrent), Onecan (Wallace)

Ketoconazole-

Ketozole (Rexcel), Nizral (Ethnor), Konazole (PCI), Hyphoral (Makers), Fungicide (Torrent), Phytoral (B & B)

Itraconazole-

Canditral (Glenmark), Sporanox (Johnson & Johnson) Fluconazole+

Tinidazole Kit-

Azostat (Crossland), V G Stat (BE), Antif-x (Twilight)

Terbinafine-

Exifine (D.R.L.), Sebifin (Glat)

(ii) Anti Protozoal & anti-amoebic-

Metronidazole-

Aristogyl (Aristo), Flagyl (Rhone-Poulenc), Metrogyl (Unique), Unimezol (Unichem), Metron (Alkem)

Furazolidone-

Fudone (Euphoric), Furoxone (S.B.)

Tinidazole-

Fasigyn (Pfizer), Tiniba (Cadila H.C.), Zoacide (Tata)

Secnidazole-

Secnil (Rhone-Poulenc), Seczol (Intas), Senizo (B.E.)

Hydroxyquinolones-

Enteroquinol (East India), Amicline (Franco India)

Combinations-

Metronidazole + Furazolidone-

Dependal-M (S.B.), Dysfur-M (B.E.)

Metronidazole + Diloxanide furoate-

Flagyl-DF (R.Poulenc), Lumigard (Sigma) Entamizole (Knoll)

Metronidazole + Nalidixic Acid-

Bacigyl (Aristo), Gramogyl (Stancare)

Tinidazole + Diloxanide furoate-

Tagrid (Core), Zoa-forte (Tata)

Tinidazole + Norfloxacin-

Diaba (Sun), Norflox TZ (Cipla), Nodd (J.K.Pharma.), Zobact (Perch)

Tinidazole + Ciprofloxacin-

Cifran CT (Ranbaxy), Ciplox TZ (Cipla), Gastrogyl (B.E.), Brakke (Francho), Ciprowin-TZ (Alembic), Strox-TZ (Dabur)

(iii) Antiviral-

Acyclovir-

Herpex (Torrent), Lovir (Eli Llly), Zovirax (Wellcome), Ocuvir (FDC), Herperax (Micronova)

Amantadine-

Amantrel (Protec)

Ribavirin-

Ribavin (Lupin)

Zidovudine-

Retrovir (Wellcome), Zidovir (Cipla)

Interferon-

Roferon-A (Piramal H.C.), Nulip (Gufic)

Lamivudine-

Lamivir (Cipla), Lamidac (Alidac)

(iv) Antileprotic-

Dapsone-

Dapsone (Wellcome)

Clofazimine-

Clofozine (Astro-IDL), Hansepran (SG Pharma)

(V) Antimalarial-

Amodiaquine-

Camoquin, Basoquin, Comaprima (Parke Davis)

Primaquine-

Malirid (IPCA), PMQ-INGA (Inga), Primaline (Unicure)

Chloroquine-

Malaquin (P.C.I.), Nivaquine-P (R. Poulenc), Resochin (Bayer)
Lariago (IPCA), Emquin (Merck).

Artesunate-

Falcigo (Cadila H.C.)

Quinine-

Qinarsol-300 (Cipla), Rubiquin (PCI)

Proguanil-

Laveran (Unicure)

Mepacrine-

Maladin (Unicure)

Pyrimethamine-

Metakelfin (Upjohn-Pharmacia), Metasulfin (PCI), Laridox (IPCA), Pyralfin (Lupin), Amalar (B & B)

Mefloquine-

MQF (Sun), Mefloc (Aristo), Confal (Lupin)

(vi) Antihelminthics and AntiInfestives-

Piperazine-

Piperazine citrate (Wellcome & Dabur), Helmacid c senna (Glaxo)

Pyrantel Pamoate-

Nemocid (IPCA), Combantrin (Pfizer), Pryanthel (Dolphin)

Diethyl Carbamazine-

Hetrazan (Wyeth), Carbamyl (Kopran), Banocide (Wellcome), Unicarbazan (Unichem).

Levamisole-

Dewormis (Glaxo), Dicaris (Ethnor), Vermisol (Khandelwal), Vizole (M.M.Labs).

Niclosamide-

Niclosan (Glaxo)

Praziquantel-

Cysticide (Merck), Distocide (V.H.B.)

Mebendazole-

Mebex (Cipla), Pantelmin (Ethnor), Wormin (Cadila)

Albendazole-

Albezole (Khandelwal), Alminth (Torrent), Bendex (Protec), Noworm (Alkem), Zentel (S.B.), Combantrin-A (Pfizer)

(vii) Antibiotics, Sulphonamides and Antituberculars-

For more details see Chapter-14

Section- B

CHAPTER- 14

Antibiotics and Sulphonamides

Chemotherapy

Chemicals have been used to treat infectious diseases for many centuries. Bacteriologists have recognised for many years that a growing culture of one micro-organism may have an inhibitory effect on the growth of another micro-organism.

Pasture and Joubert in 1877 observed that certain air-borne bacteria were capable of inhibiting the growth of anthrox bacilli. By this time many chemicals were known which eradicated infection when applied topically as antiseptic and disinfectants, but these were too toxic for systemic administration.

The anti-infective drug treatment of systemic infections was put on a rational basis in 1906 by the "Father of Chemotherapy", the famous German chemist Paul Ehrlich. In 1928 Alexander Flamming noted that some colonies of Staphylococci were lysed when the medium was contaminated by a mould (genus, Penicillium notatum) and called it Penicillin

The modern era of Chemotherapy of infections began with the clinical use of Sulphonamide in 1936. The golden age of antimicrobial therapy started with the production of antibiotic Penicillin in 1941, when it first become available for limited clinical trials.

Originally the term Chemotherapy was applied only to the use of synthetic chemicals employed to treat infectious disease. But the current usage makes no distinction between antibiotics and chemotherapeutic agents of synthetic origin.

"Chemotherapy" is a term that applies to both natural and synthetic chemicals used in a manner intended to interfere with the functioning of foreign cell populations.

Antibiotics

"Antibiotics" are chemical compounds produced by living micro-organisms and are capable of inhibiting or killing bacteria and other micro-oganisms.

Antibacterial Spectrum

The antimicrobials are generally described in term of their range of activity or spectrum over various pathogenic micro-organisms.

The antibiotics are often classified as:

(i) Narrow Spectrum Antibiotic e.g. Penicillin, Erythromycin, Lincomycin, etc.

(ii) Broad Spectrum Antibiotics e.g. Tetracyclines, Ampicillin, Cephalexin, Ciprofloxacin, etc.

Modes of Action of Antimicrobial Agents

Primarily, the modes of action of antimicrobial agents are

(1) Bacteriostatic action

It is the ability of a compound to inhibit the growth & multiplication of the invading micro-organisms, while the body's own defence mechanism destroys them, e.g. Erythromycin, Sulphonamides, Trimethoprim, etc.

(2) Bactericidal action

It means an actual killing effect on the invading micro-organisms, e.g. Penicillins, Cephalosporins, Aminoglycosides,etc.

In high doses some of the bacteriostatic agents exerts bactericidal action.

Most of the commonly used antimicrobial agents act by one of the following basic mechanisms

(i) Inhibition of bacterial cell wall synthesis, e.g. Penicillins, Cephalosporins, Cycloserine, Vancomycin, etc.

(ii) Inhibition of cytoplasmic membrane function. e.g. Polymyxin-B, Colistin, Nystatin, Pamphotericin, etc.

(iii) Inhibition of protein synthesis e.g. Streptomycin, Gentamycin, Tobramycin, Tetracylines, Macrolides, etc.

(iv) Substrate competition (PABA) with essential metabolite. e.g. Sulphonamides, Trimethoprim.

(v) Inhibition of nucleic acid synthesis. e.g. Nalidix acid,

Ciprofloxacin, Rifampicin, Ethambutol, various anticancer agents, etc.

Potency

The potency of an antimicrobial agent is usually expressed on the basis of minimum inhibitory concentration (M.I.C.) at which it is capable of inhibiting the multiplication of the susceptible micro-organisms.

Slective Toxicity

It is the ability of chemicals to strike slectively at foreign cells, without causing significant damage to the host cells.

Bacterial Resistance

Bacterial resistance is a major medical problem that limits the usefulness of many antibiotics. Considered by species, bacteria are susceptible to some antibiotics are resistant to others. But bacterial strain may develop resistance to antimicrobial agents which are supposed to be normally effective against that species.

The bacteria which is resistant to one antimicrobial agent are found to be resistant to a second drug without having been exposed to the latter, is known as "Cross Resistance". It is more common among closely chemically related drugs and between drugs having same modes of action or attachment.

The bacterial resistance to antimicrobial agents can be natural or acquired.

Classification of Antibiotics

The antibiotics can be classified according to their :

(a) Source- The sources of the antibiotics can be Fungi (e.g. Penicillin from Penicillium notatum and others), or Actinomycetes (e.g. Tetracycline from Streptomyces rimosus and others), or Bacteria (e.g. Polymyxins from Bacillus polymyxa and others)

(b) Chemical nature- According to chemical nature the antibiotics can be containing - one aminoacid (e.g. Chloramphenicol), two amino acids (e.g. Penicillins), Polypeptides (e.g. Polymyxin) and can be Aminoglycoside (e.g. Gentamicin), Polyene (e.g. Nystatin), containing macrocyclic lactone ring (e.g. Erythromycin) and misc. compounds.

(c) Mode of action- The antibiotics which inhibit cell wall

synthesis, or inhibit protein synthesis, or inhibit cytoplasmic membrane function, or inhibit nucleic acid synthesis.

(d) Antibacterial Spectrum- According to antibacterial spectrum the antibiotics can be narrow spectrum antibiotics or broad spectrum antibiotics.

Adverse Effects of Antimicrobial Agents

The adverse effects of antimicrobials fall into the following three general classes:

(i) Direct toxic effects upon such organs as liver, kidneys, G.I. tract, or the optic, auditory & other peripheral nerves. For examples Aminoglycosides, Polymyxins, Cephaloridine may exert nephrotoxic effect, Chloramphenicol, Erythromycin may exert hepatotoxic effects and neurotoxicity may occurs with Streptomycin, etc.

(ii) Allergic reactions and other types of hypersensitivity reactions affecting the skin, bone marrow, circulating blood and other structures. For example hypersensitivity reactions (anaphylactic shock) cases have often been reported with inj. Penicillin.

(iii) Superinfections are a result of drug induced overgrowth by resistant bacterias or fungi. This may be the result of an indiscriminate use of antibiotics. For example prolonged use of Tetracyclines may cause Vit. B-complex deficiency in the body due to the alteration of the normal intestinal bacterial flora.

Few Common Antibiotics

(A) Narrow - Spectrum Penicillins

(1) Penicillin- It is the first antibiotic used in man. The Penicillin inhibits bacterial cell wall systhesis and there by exerts bactericidal action.

The Penicillin is used in all pyogenic coccal infections caused by Gram+ve & Gram-ve cocci, in Gram+ve & Gram-ve bacilli infections, in Spirochetes & Actinomycetes infections. Its mode of uses are parenteral I.M. inj; oral and topical applications.

Common Penicillin Preparations

Benzyl Penicillin, Procaine Penicillin, Benzathine Penicillin & Phenoxymethyl Penicillin preparations are available in the market.

Injections- Bistrepen (Alembic), Crys-4 (Sarabhai), Dicrysticin-S

(Sarabhai), Fortified P.P.(Sarabhai), Longacillin (HAL), Penidure (Wyeth)

Oral- Crystapen V granules (Glaxo), Kaypen (HAL), Pentids (Sarabhai)

Untoward Effects of Penicillin

The Penicillins are among the least toxic of antibiotics. Occasional incidence of hypersensitivity to the Penicillins (from minor allergic states to serious anaphylactic shocks) has been seen in about 1% to 5% cases.

The Penicillins are ineffective against Penicillinase-producing organisms.

(2) Cloxacillin- Cloxacillin is a semi-synthetic Penicillin which is unaffected by "Penicillinase enzyme" liberated by certain bacteria.

It is acid-stable and is effectively absorbed after oral administration, but can also be given parenterally. When given orally on an empty stomach 1 gm. of Cloxacillin achieve a peak plasma level of 5-10 mcg/ ml in one hour. It is conta-indicated in patients having hypersensitivity to Penicillin.

Few Cloxacillin preparations available in the market are:

Bioclox (Biochem), Clocilin (PCI), Klox (lyka).

Ampilox (Biochem), Ampoxin (Unichem), Megapen (Aristo), Duoclox (FDC), Synerpen (Bombay Tab.), Ducidal (Obsurge), Dynaclox (Micro), Symbiotic (Lesante)

Nataclox (Sun), Novaclox (Cipla), Mytimox (Panacea), Suprimox (Rexcel).

(B) Broad Spectrum Penicillins

(1) Ampicillin- Ampicillin is a semi-synthetic Penicillin with broad-spectrum bactericidal activity. Ampicillin is amphoteric and therefore ionized at all pHs, resulting in poor & slow oral absorption. The presence of food in the stomach further delays absorption. An oral dose of 500 mg produces peak levels of about 3 mcg/ ml in 2 hours. Within 6 hours of administration about 30% of the dose is excreted, mostly unchanged in the urine.

Ampicillin is mainly indicated in the treatment of infections caused by Streptococci, non-penicillinase producing Staphylococci, Pneumococci, Meningococci, Gonococci, E-coli, H. influenzae, Salmonella and Proteus species.

It is contra-indicated in patients having hypersensitivity to Penicillin. Used orally as capsule , kid -tab, syrup & drops and also as injection.

Few Ampicillin preparations available in the market are:

Albercilin (Hoechst), Bacipen (Alembic), Biocilin (Biochem), Roscillin (Ranbaxy)

Ampilong (American Remd.), Prompicin (Geno), Ampilin (Lyka), Aristocillin (Aristo)

Ampitum (FDC), Sulbacin (Unichem), Ampilin-SB (Lyka).

(2) *Amoxycillin-* Amoxycillin is a derivative of Ampicillin and has a similar antibacterial spectrum. It is more potent & effective than Ampicillin in a lesser dose against Streptococci faecalis and Salmonella species. It also penetrates purulent and mucoid bronchial secretions more effectively than Ampicillin.

Its advantage over Ampicillin are that for comparable oral doses Amoxycillin achieve app. twice the serum concentrations, the presence of food in the stomach does not greatly interfere with absorption. An oral dose of 250 mg produces peak levels of 4 mcg/ml in 2 hours. The usual adult dose is 250 mg 8 hourly and 60% is excreted unchanged in the urine.

Amoxycillin is also ineffective in infections caused by Penicillin-resistant organisms and is contra-indicated in patients having hypersensitivity to Penicillin. The incidence of particulary diarrhoea with Amoxycillin is 70% less than with Ampicillin. Used orally as capsule, kid-tab, syrup, drops and also as injection.

Few Amoxycillin preparations available in the market are:

Blumox (Blue Cross), Hipen (Cadila H.C.), Lamoxy (Lyka), Mox (Rexcel), Moxydil (Duphar), Amoxil (German Remedies), Natamox (Natco), Wymox (Wyeth), Carbomox (Win-Medicare), Cidoresp (Roussel), Moxycarb (Nicholas), Bulmox-BH (Blue Cross), Bromolin (Protec), Respimox (Wockhardt),Moxene (Twilight), Augmentin (S.B.), Clavam (Alkem), Nuclav (Knoll), Moxclav (Rexcel)

(3) *Carbenicillin-* It is a semi-synthetic broad spectrum Penicillin, mainly used for treating Pseudomonas & Proteus species infections and certain Gram negative organisms. It is not absorbed when given by mouth and has to be administered parenterally.

It is excreted almost entirely in the urine. Its side effects include hypokalaemia and alteration in platelet function with spontaneous bleeding.

Few Carbenicillin brands available in the market are:

Biopence (Biochem), Carbelin (Lyka), Pyopen (German Remedies).

(C) Macrolides

The Macrolides antibiotics structurally consist of a large lactone ring to which sugars are attached. They include Erythromycin, Oleandomycin, Spiramycin, Roxithromycin, Azithromycin, etc.

The antibacterial spectrum is almost similar to Penicillin though little broader. They are primarily effective against Gram positive cocci, Bacteroides fragilis, Corynebacterium diptheriae, H.influenzae, M. Pneumoniae, Chlamydia, Neisseriae, Brucellae, Spirochetes and some Rickettsiae. They exert bacteriostatic effect, but in high concentrations exert bactericidal effect. G.I. disturbances and allergy being the commonest adverse reactions with Macrolides.

Few Macrolides preparations available in the market are:

(i) Erythromycin- Althrocin (Alembic), E-mycin (Themis Ph.), Erythrocin (Abbott), Eltocin (IPCA), Eroate (Lupin), Ero-B (Lupin).

(ii) Spiramycin- Rovamycin (Rhone - Poulenc)

(iii) Roxithromycin- Roxibid (Cadila Ph.), Roxid (Alembic), Rulide (Roussel)

(iv) Azithromycin- Azithral (Alembic), Aziwok (Wockhardt), Azolide (J.K.Ph.)

(v) Clarithromycin- Claribid (Abbott), Clarithro (Alembic), Celex (Glaxo), Clarimac (Cadila-H), Anaclar (Twilight)

(D) Lincosamides

The Lincosamide antibiotics, Lincomycin and Clindamycin, are similar to the macrolides regarding their antibacterial spectrum, mode of action and therapeutic applications. They are usually well tolerated, but may cause fatal colitis. This has restricted their use to a few specific and serious infections in hospitalized patients.

(i) Lincomycin- Lincocin (Upjohn), Lynx (Wallace)

(ii) Clindamycin- Dalcap (Unisearch), Dalacin (Pharmacia)

(E) Tetracyclines

The Tetracyclines are a group of drugs that have a similar antibiotic action, though they differ some what in their pharmacology. The Tetracyclines have a broad antibacterial spectrum which covers Gram positive & Gram negative bacteria, Rickettsiae, Mycoplasma, Treponema pallidum and Chlamydia. They are not effective against Tubercle bacillus, Pseudomonas and Proteus.

The oral Tetracyclines exert a bacteriostatic effect, however higher concentrations or parenteral administration may exert a bactericidal effect.

Forms of Tetracyclines commonly used are:

(i) Tetracycline Hydrochloride- Hostacycline (Hoechst), Resteclin (Sarabhai), Subamycin (Day's), Threocycline (IDPL)

(ii) Demeclocycline- Ledermycin (Wyeth)

(iii) Oxytetracycline- Terramycin, Terramycin SF (Pfizer)

(iv) Doxycycline- Doxypal (Jagson Pal), Doxy-1 (USV), Laa (Bombay Tab.), Martidox (Walter Bushnell), Vibazine DT (Pfizer).

(F) Chloramphenicol

It is a broad spectrum bacteriostatic antibiotic and inhibits bacterial protein systhesis in susceptible organisms. Chloramphenicol is a potent, potentially toxic antibiotic which should be reserved for the treatment of life threatening infections particularly, Typhoid Fever, H. influenzae or K. Pneumoniae infections. It is also useful for the treatment of bacterial conjunctivitis.

Its disadvantages includes, chances of development of haematological abnormalities (e.g. aplastic anaemia), Grey body syndrome in newborn babies and hypersensitivity reactions. It is used orally as capsule, syrup/ suspension, injection and topical application.

Few Chloramphenicol brands are :

Chlormycetin (Parke Davis), Enteromycetin (Dey's), Paraxin (Nicholas-Piramal), Reclor (Sarabhai), Kemicetine (Mac)

(G) Cephalosporins

The Cephalosporins include a group of useful antibiotics having broad spectrum, bactericidal activity. The antibiotics of this group share a peptide nucleus, 7 amino cephalosproanic acid

(7-ACA), resembling that of the Penicillins. They also act similarly in that they prevent cross-link formation in the mucopeptide of the bacterial cell wall by inhibiting a transpectidase.

The Cephalosporins are highly effective against most of the Gram + ve organisms like Staphylococcus (including Penicillin resistant penicillinase producing Staph. aureus), Streptococcus, Pneumococcus, Corynebacteria, Treponema pallidum, Clostrida, Listeria monocytogenes and Bacillus anthracis. These are also effective against many Gram - ve organisms like H. influenzae, E-coli, Gonococcus, Meningococcus, Salmonella, Shigella, Treponema pallidum and Klebsilla. But these are not effective against Tubercle bacillus, Pseudomonas, Bacteroides, Bordetella, Virus and Fungi.

The main adverse reaction of the Cephalosporins is hypersensitivity (including anaphylactic shock), allergy and nephrotoxicity (in large dose).

The available Cephalosporins are administered by various routes as written below:

(i) Oral Cephalosporins

Cephalexin- Ceff (Lupin), Neocef (Allenburys), Phexin (Glaxo), Sporidex (Ranbaxy), Carbicef (Sun), Resporidex (Stancare), Cefalong (American Remd), Nufex (R.P.G.), Alexin (Dabur)

Cefadroxil- Cefadrox (Aristo), Droxyl (Torrent), Odoxil (Lupin), Vepan (Indoco), Cefadur (Protec), BID (Kopran), Kefloxin (Solus)

Cefaclor- Distaclor (Eli lilly), Keflor (Ranbaxy).

Cefixime- Cefspan (Wellcome), Topcef (Torrent), Taxim-O (Alkem)

(ii) Parenteral Cephalosporins

Cephaloridine- Cephaxin Inj. (Biochem), Ceporan (Glaxo).

Cefazolin- Alcizon (Alembic), Orizolin (Alidac), Reflin (Ranbaxy), Azolin (Biochem), Cezolin (Lupin)

Ceftizoxime- Cefizox (Wellcome), Epocelin (Rallis).

Cefotaxime- Omnatax (Hoechst), Omnicef (Aristo), Taxim (Alkem).

Ceftriaxone sod.- Monocef (Aristo), Monotax (Biochem), Zefone (Indo Pharma), Oframax (Ranbaxy), Nosocef (Merind), Taxone (Mapra)

Ceftazidime- Ceftidin (Lyka), Fortum (Glaxo), Orzid (Orchid)

Cefoperazone- Lorizon (Dolphin), Magnamycin (Pfizer), Myticef (Panacea).

(iii) Oral & Parenteral Cephalosporins

Cefuroxime- Ceftum (Allenburys), Furoxil (Torrent), Supacef (Glaxo), Zocef (Alkem)

(H) Quinolones (Fluroquinolone)

The Fluroquinolones include a group of broad-spectrum, bactericidal antibiotics. They act by inhibiting the enzyme (DNA Gyrase) responsible for supercoiling the DNA strands during bacterial replication.

The Fluroquinolones are highly effective against penicillinase and beta-lactamase producing organisms, methicillin resistant Staphylococci, E-coli, Klebsiella, Proteus, Pseudomonas, Salmonella typhosa, Streptococcus, Gonococcus & Shigella species.

The Quinolones preparations available in the market are:

Nalidixic Acid- Gramoneg (Ranbaxy), Negadix (CFL), Ulix-P (Blue Cross).

Norfloxacin-Norbactin (Rexcel), Norbid (Alembic), Norflox (Cipla).

Ciprofloxacin- Alcipro (Alkem), Cifran (Ranbaxy), Ciplox (Cipla), Ciprobid (Cadila H.C.), Strox (Dabur), Quintor (Torrent), Zoxan (FDC).

Pefloxacin- Pelox (Wockhardt), Qucin (Aristo), Pfen (Bombay Tab.), Proflox (Protec), Pefcin (Torrent), Rolox (Recon)

Lomefloxacin- Lomflox-400 (IPCA), Lomibact (TDPL), Qumax (Alkem).

Ofloxacin- Tarivid (Hoechst), Zanocin (Stancare), Zenflox (Mankind)

Sparfloxacin- Rexpar (Ranbaxy), Sparlox (Sun), Sparquin (Aristo).

(I) Aminoglycosides

The aminoglycosides are composed of amino sugar connected by glycoside linkage. All aminoglycosides are bactericidal (except Streptomycin which may be bactericidal in higher dose or bacteriostatic) and active against Gram + ve and mainly Gram - ve organisms including E-coli, Klebsiella, Pseudomonas,

Proteus, Aerobactor, Shigella & Salmonella, Streptomycin and Kanamycin are also active against Mycobacterium tuberculosis, while Gentamicin, Amikacin & Tobramycin are active against Streptococcus faecalis and Pseudomonas aeruginos. Bacteria frequently develop parmanent resistance to Aminoglycosides.

The Aminoglycosides inhibit bacterial protein synthesis. As they are poorly absorbed following oral administration, they have to be given by injection and/or as topical preparations.

Main untoward side-effets of Aminoglycosides include the possibility of toxic effect on the eighth cranial nerves (ototoxicity) and to a lesser degree, nephrotoxicity and neuro-muscular blockade.

Forms of Aminoglycosides commonly used are:

Streptomycin- Ambistryn-S (Sarabhai), Streptomycin (Alembic).

Kanamycin- Kancin (Alembic), Kanamycin (Biochem), Kanamac (Macleods).

Gentamicin- G10/20/40/60/80 (Kee Pharma), Garamycin (Fulford), Genticyn (Nicholas), Merigenta (Mercury), Gen (Mac)

Amikacin- Amicin (Biochem), Amitax (Alkem), Ivimicin (FDC), Mikacin (Aristo).

Netilmicin- Netromycin (Fulford).

Tobramycin- Tobacin (Aristo), Tobraneg (Eli lilly).

Sisomicin- Ensamycin (Fulford), Sisoptin (Merind).

Neomycin- Cap. Neomycin sulphate (Unichem), Nebasulf skin oint & powder (Omni-Protech), Neosporin powder (Wellcome).

(J) Polymyxins & Colistin

Polymyxins are cyclic polypetides, all differing in their amino acid content & obtained from Bacillus polymyxa. Polymyxin-B Sulphate has therapeutic value among Polymyxins.

Polymyxin-B has a narrow spectrum limited to action against gram - ve organisms (except Proteus & Neisseria), with bactericidal activity. It is usually administered topically & rarely oral, I.V. or intrathecal administration is warranted.

Colistin is a bactericidal polypeptide antibiotic, obtained from Bacillus colistinus and has an antibacterial spectrum & mode of action similar to that of Polymyxin-B, but is less potent . It is avilable as Colistin Sulphate for oral use.

Polymyxin-B- Aerosporin Inj. (Wellcome), Andresporin drops (Andre).

Colistin Sulphate- Walamycin (Wallace), Colistop (Indipharma)

Sulphonamides

The Sulphonamides were the first effective Chemotherapeutic agents to be employed systemically for the prevention and cure of bacterial infections in man. The Sulphonamides have a basic chemical resemblance to Para-Amino Benzoic Acid (PABA). They are white crystalline powders mostly poorly soluble in water and having bacteriostatic activites.

The Sulphonamides have a broad-spectrum antimicrobial activity against both gram + ve and gram - ve micro-organisms and some Protozoa, including-group A Streptococci , H. influenzae, H. ducreyi, Pneumococci, E-coli, Cornybacterium, Cheolera vibrio, Pasturella pestis, Bacillus anthracis, Actinomycetes, Meningococci, Shigellae & Chlamydia trachomatis, Klebsiella, Enterobacter & Proteus may be sensitive to very high concentrations. Several species of Staphylococci, Enterococci, Clostridium and Pseudomonas are highly resistant to Sulphonamides. The Sulphonamides (Sulfadoxine) are an effective adjunct to Pyrimethamine in treating malaria.

The Sulphonamide are structurally analogues & competitive antagonists of PABA, and thus prevent the normal bacterial utilization of PABA for the synthesis of Folic acid. Folic acid derivatives are essential for purine and ultimately DNA synthesis in bacteria. Specifically the Sulphonamides competitively inhibit the enzyme dihydrofolic acid synthetase and there by prevent dihydrofolic acid formation (PABA is the normal substrate for the enzyme). This reaction is closely related to the concentration of the Sulfa drugs & PABA.

The Sulfa drugs (excepting the Sulphaguanidine) are well absorbed from the G.I. tract (app. 70 to 100% of oral dose) and become bound to protein and to some extent are acetylated. They are excreted mainly through the Kidneys. Acetylation mainly occur in the liver. Each Sulpha drug is acetylated to different extent. It is toxic in nature and has no antibacterial activity and are poorly soluble in urine and are likely to produce crystalluria.

Based on the absorption and excretion patterns, the Sulphonamides can be classified as:

(i) Short-acting Sulphonanides e.g. Sulphacetamide, Sulphadiazine and Sulphadimidine group

(ii) Intermediate-acting Sulphonamides e.g. Sulphamethoxazole & Sulphamoxole.

(iii) Long-acting Sulphonamides e.g. Sulphadimethoxine and Sulphamethoxy pyridazine.

(iv) Ultra-long acting Sulphonamides e.g. Sulphametoprazine & Sulfadoxine (used in combination with Pyrimethamine for the treatment of malaria).

The Sulpha drugs are usually administered orally (Tablet, Suspension), occasionally intravenously, rarely subcutaneously and topically.

The allergic skin rashes are fairly frequent complications of Sulpha therapy. Crystalluria can occur and may cause irritation, haematuria, renal colic, anuria & fatal uraemia. The Sulpha therapy may also cause agranulocytosis, thrombocytopenia, or aplastic anaemia.

The Sulpha drugs may produce kernicterus in the foetus and neonate. Their use is not advisable in infants & young children.

Co-trimoxazole

The generic name Co-trimoxazole is used for Sulphamethoxazole 400 mg and Trimethoprim 80 mg. per tablet. The above combination product has proved to be very useful antimicrobial drug. Trimethoprim is chemically related to Pyrimethamine an older antimalarial compound and is 20 to 100 times more potent than Sulphamethoxazole. Sulphamethoxazole is absorbed and excreted at about the same rate as Trimethoprim. The antibacterial spectrum of Trimethoprim is similar to that of Sulphamethoxazole.

Mode of Action

The antimicrobial activity of Trimethoprim and Sulphamethoxazole results from the action on two sequential steps of the enzymatic pathway for the synthesis of Tetrahydrofolic acid (Folinic acid). The Sulphonamides being structurally related to Para-aminobenzoic acid (PABA) act by competitive blockade of the enzyme Dihydrofolic acid synthetase, necessary for the conversion of PABA to Dihydrofolic acid.

Trimethoprim interferes with the action of Dihydrofolic acid reductase, an enzyme which converts Dihydrofolic acid to Tetrahydrofolic acid, an essential stage in the bacterial purine, and ultimately DNA synthesis.

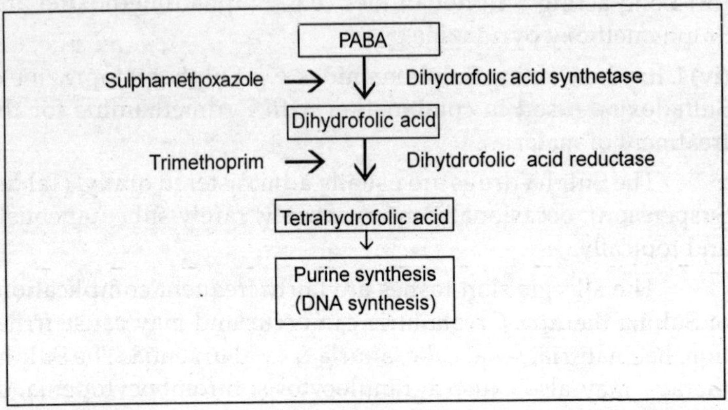

Fig.26

Absorption of Co-trimoxazole by oral route is rapid, peak plasma levels occur between 2 to 4 hours after administration and detectable amount have been found after 24 hours. Individually both Trimethoprim and Sulphamethoxazole are bacteriostatic, but their combination is said to have bactericidal effect.

The available Sulphonamides preparations in the market are:

Sulphadiazine- Sulphadiazine (Rhone-Poulenc).

Sulphadimethoxine- Madribon (Rhone-Poulenc).

Sulphacetamide- Drops-Albucid (Nicholas), Locula (East India).

Sulfamoxole- Sulfuno (German Remedies).

Co-trimazine- Aubril (Ciba), Silizine (B.E.), Triglobe (Astra-IDL). (Trimethoprim + Sulphadiazine)

Co-trimoxazole- Bactrim (Piramal H.C.), Colizole (East India), Kombina (Deys), Oriprim (Cadila H.C.), Sepmax & Septran (Wellcome), Synastat (Roussel), Rizol (Bombay Tab.), Servoprim (Hoechest), Ciplin (Cipla), Trim Forte (Alkem), Supristol (G-Remedies), Duocidal (Kr.Anti), Otrim (Biochem), Sumertrol (Themis Ch.)

Section- B

CHAPTER - 15

Anti-Tuberculous Drugs

Tuberculosis is generally a chronic infection caused by Mycobacterium tuberculosis, and occasionally by Mycobacterium bovis. Mycobacterium tuberculosis is a bacillus that can remain dormant in the human host for years.

Infection of the upper lung is the most common form of tuberculosis and occurs in majority of cases in the middleaged and elderly patients, usually originate from the reactivation of a dormant lesion. The acute systemic non-pulmonary forms of the disease like Tuberculosis Adenitis (affecting the lymph, glands), Tuberculosis Peritonitis (affecting the peritoneum), Gastro-intestinal Tuberculosis (affecting the G.I. tract-usually causing ulcers), Tuberculosis Meningitis (affecting the meninges of the brain), Tuberculosis Pericarditis (affecting the pericardium), Tuberculosis Osteomyelitis (affecting bones & joints) and acute Miliary Tuberculosis (a very acute & toxic generalised condition) are encountered in the lower socio-economic groups of society where malnutrition, poor hygiene, overcrowded living conditions and substandard medical facilities prevail.

Clinically, Tuberculosis, presents no special symptoms, except those that indicate the infection of the involved organ. Acute Miliary Tuberculosis may present as a systemic febrile illness.

Classification

The antituberculous drugs are classified generally on the basis of their efficacy and safety. They are divided into two major groups:

(1) Primary Drugs- The primary drugs or the "first-line" drugs are used in standard therapeutic regimens, due to their high level of

efficacy and least toxicity .The majority of the patients are treated sucessfully with these drugs. The primary drugs are Isoniazid (INH), Rifampicin, Ethambutol, Streptomycin.

(2) Secondary Drugs- The secondary drugs or the "second-line" drugs (alternative drugs) are used occasionally because of bacterial resistance or certain patient-related factors. The secondary drugs are -Pyrazinamide, Ethionamide, PAS (Para-aminosalicyclic acid), Cyclosrine, Viomycin, Thiacetazone, Thiocarlide, Kanamycin, Amikacin, Capreomycin.

Some authorities consider PAS as a primary drug when it is used in children and as a secondary drug for adults.

Common Anti-Tuberculous Drugs

(a) Isoniazid (INH)

The Isoniazid is the most effective, most economical drug for the treatment of Tuberculosis, as it is least toxic & most efficacious. It exerts both tuberculostatic and tuberculocidal effects. The tuberculocidal effect is exerted only against actively growing Tubercle bacilli.

INH is taken orally and after absorption from the gut, diffuses well into the body tissues, including the CNS and excerted primarily through the Kidneys. INH also penetrates into macrophages so that it is effective against intracellular Tubercle bacilli.

The INH is relatively free from side effects in doses not exceeding 300 mg. daily. It may cause restlessness, insomnia, nausea, vomiting, peripheral neuritis and muscle twitching, which can be pervented by the use of Pyridoxine (Vit.-B_6) 10-20 mg. daily.

Few INH brands avilable in the market are:

Isokin (Parke-Davis), Isonex (Pfizer), Solonex (Macleods), Inapas (Neo Pharma), Siozide (Albert David), Erbazide (Mac), Unithiben (Unichem)

(b) Rifampicin

Rifampicin is a semisysnthetic derivative of Rifamycin B. It is considered to be the most potent anti T.B. drug available. Rifampicin has a broad-spectrum of activity and inhibits the growth of many Gam + ve cocci, Gram - ve bacteria such as E-coli, Pseudomonas, Klebsiella, Proteus and Anaerobes. It is also highly effective against Mycobacterium tuberculosis and many atypical Mycobacteria.

Rifampicin is well absorbed on oral administration and exerts bactericidal action. It acts by inhibiting bacterial DNA-dependent RNA polymerase and thereby interferes with RNA synthesis. It is metabolized by deacetylation and is excreted mainly in the bile and less than 10% as unchanged in the urine.

The usual does is 600 mg. orally (for adults above 50 kg. weight) given once daily, either 1 hour before or 2 hours after a meal. Rifampicin does not cause untoward effects when given in usual doses. Liver damage, renal failure, shock and thrombocytopenic purpura may occur. The drug should be used with caution in alcoholics and patients with hepatic disease.

Few Rifampicin brands available in the market are :

R-cin (Lupin), Rifaminal (Alembic), Rimactane (Novartis), Zucox (Glaxo), Rifacilin (PCI), Macox (Macleods), Cavidin (Merind), Ticin (Themis)

Rifampicin + Isoniazid- Anticox (Unichem), Rcinex (Lupin), Macox Plus (Macleods), Rifaminal Forte (Alembic), Rimactazid (Novartis), Zucox Plus (Glaxo).

(c) Ethambutol

Ethambutol is a synthetic drug used as a first line drug in the treatment of Tuberculosis. It is a bacteriostatic agent, possibly depressing RNA synthesis and effectively inhibiting strains which are resistant to INH or Streptomycin.

Ethambutol is well absorbed on oral administration and the absorption is not affected by the presence of food in the stomach. It is excreted unchanged about 80% in the urine.

Ethambutol produces very few adverse reactions in daily doses of 15 mg/kg. In high doses it may cause toxic damage of the optic nerve (loss of visual activity due to optic neuritis and loss of colour vision), allergic drug reaction (rashes, pruritis), joint pains, abdominal pain, hallucinations and peripheral neuropathy.

Few Ethambutol brands available in the market are :

Combutol (Lupin), Myambutol (Wyeth), Mycobutol (Cadila Ph.), Themibutol (Themis Chem.), Ecox (Macleods), Koxi (Plethico) Ethambutol + INH- Combunex (Lupin), Myconex (Cadila). Themibutol Plus (Themis Ch.)

Ethambutol + INH + Rifampicin- AKT - 3 (Lupin)

(d) Streptomycin

It is an antibiotic and bactericidal in-vitro, where as, in-vivo it is essentially suppressing the growth of the Tubercle bacillus. Streptomycin is used in combination with other primary drugs in the treatment of Tuberculosis, specially in patients with impaied liver function. The usual dose is 1g. IM daily.

Allergic reaction (Skin rashes) may sometimes occur, ototoxicity (Vestibular mainly) and nephrotoxicity are related to dosage and duration of therapy, specially in the elderly patients and those with renal insufficiency.

Few Streptomycin brands available in the market are :

Inj. Ambistryn - S (Sarabhai), Merstrep (Merind), Streptomycin (Alembic).

(e) Pyrazinamide

It is chemically related to Nicotinamide. Pyrazinamide reaches the C.S.F. in high concentration and possesses bactericidal action against Mycobacterium tuberculosis. It is readily absorbed on oral administration and widely distributed throughout the body tissues. The usual dose is 20-30 mg./kg./ day orally with a maximum of 3 g. daily.

Hepatotoxicity is the most common untoward effect. Other adverse effects are possibility of nausea, vomiting, anorexia, arthralgia, urticaria, fever and diabetes mellitus. It is contraindicated in gout, hepatic dysfunction and diabetes mellitus.

Few Pyrazinamide preparations are listed below :

Copyrazin (PCI), Macrozide (Macleods), P-zide (Cadila), PZA-Ciba (Novartis), Rizap (Glaxo), Tibimide (Themis), Pyzina (Lupin), Piraldina (Pharmed)

Pyrazinamide + INH + Rifampicin- Anticox - Z Kit (Unichem), ISO Rifazin (PCI), Macox-ZH (Macleods), Rcinex- Z (Lupin), Rimactazid + Z (Novartis), Tricox (Themis Chem), Zucox Kit (Glaxo)

Pyrazinamide + INH + Rifampicin + Ethambutol- 4D (Novartis), AKT-4 (Lupin), Anticox-4 (Unichem), CX-5 (Cadila H.C.), Forecox (Macleods), Themicox -4 Kit (Themis Chem), Zucox-E Kit (Glaxo).

(f) Ethionamide

Ethionamide suppresses the multiplication of human strain of M. tuberculosis and is used for the treatment of Tuberculosis resistant to first-line drugs . It is rapidly absorbed from the gut and is widely distributed in the C.S.F. as well. The usual dose is 0.5-1g orally daily in divided doses or as a single dose at night.

Adverse reactions are G.I. disturbances, including metallic taste, depression, insomnia, convulsions, rashes, menorrhagia, gynaecomastia, impotence, peripheral neuritis, optic neuritis, hepatotoxicity and hypothyroidism may occur. It is contraindicated in hepatic dysfunction & hypersensitive cases.

Few Ethionamide brands available in the market are:

Ethide (Lupin), Ethiocid (Themis), Myobid (Panacea), Ethomid (Macleods)

(g) Prothionamide

Prothionamide is similar in its action, use,dosage and toxicity to Ethionamide. Prothicid (Themis), Protomid (Macleods), Mycotuf-P (Lesante) are the brands of Prothionamide available in the market.

(h) Cycloserine

Cycloserine is a broad - spectrum antibiotic, acts by inhibiting cell wall synthesis. Cycloserine is used in combination with other effective agents to treat Tuberculosis resistant to first-line drugs. It is rapidly absorbed from the gut & widely distributed in the body tissues and enters the C.S.F. The usual dose is 0.5 - 1gm./ day orally in divided doses.

Adverse reactions are tremors, dysarthria, vertigo, confusion, seizures, headache, psychotic states and causes Vit. B_{12} / Folic acid deficiency. Cycloserine is the most toxic of the second-line drugs. It is contraindicated in epilepsy, depression, psychotic states, alcoholism, renal failure and hypersensitivity.

Few Cycloserine brands available in the market are:

Cyclorine (Lupin), Myser (Panacea), Coxerin (Macleods), Cyserine (V.H.B.)

Chemotherapeutic Regimens

For the treatment of Tuberculosis there is no general agreement on an optimal regimen or duration of treatment. Both Pulmonary and Extra-Pulmonary disease must always be treated with multiple drugs. The treatment of Tuberculosis may be divided into two phases :-

(1) Initial Phase- The simultaneous of at least 3 drugs-INH and Rifampicin, with Ethambutol or Streptomycin. These drugs should be continued for 8 weeks.

(2) Continuation Phase- After the initial phase, treatment is continued with only 2 drugs, one of which should be INH (Provided it is not contraindicated), with Rifampicin, Ethambutol or Streptomycin.

Sufficient data are now available on the outcome of treatment with initial phase followed by continuation phase, which confirms that a course of 9 months duration gives satisfactory results in Pulmonary T.B. and a total treatment period of 12 months in Extra-Pulmonary T.B.

Short-course therapy is now commonly used and the regimen is in initial phase of 4 drugs - INH, Rifampicin, Pyrazinamide and Streptomycin for about 8 weeks, followed by twice-weekly Streptomycin, INH and Rifampicin for the continuation phase, till a total treatment time of 6 months.

The main objective of using such regimen is to prevent the emergence of drug resistant Tubercle bacillus, which is a therapeutic problem.

Section- B

CHAPTER- 16

Analgesics and Antipyretics

Pain

It is an unpleasant sensation felt when impulses of noxious stimuli are transmitted to the brain through nerve fibres.

Pain Receptors

The pain receptors are free nerve endings. Superficial layers of the skin, periosteum, the joint surfaces, the arterial walls and certain parts of the meninges are well supplied with such nerve endings.

There are two types of pain fibres which carry signals from various parts of the body to the spinal cord are:

(a) A-delta fibres- They are small, myelinated & carry pain signals at a faster pace.

(b) C-delta fibres- They are very small, unmyelinated & carry pain signals slower than A-delta fibres.

Most of the internal organs and tissues are supplied with C-delta fibres, where as the skin is supplied with both types of pain receptors.

Factors Stimulating Pain Receptors

The factors stimulating pain receptors are Mechanical, Thermal (hot or cold) and Chemicals (include-Acids, Potassium ions, Acetylcholine, Proteolytic enzymes, Histamine, Serotonin, Bradykinin and Prostaglandins).

The pain receptors donot get adapted to the pain stimuli, rather they will continue to transmit pain impulses as long as the pain stimulus continues.

Pathway of Pain Receptors

The pain impulses from the different parts of the body are first transmitted to the spinal cord, from where they are carried to the brain.

Perception of the pain is probably a function of the "Thalamus" and the "Cerebral Cortex" is believed to play a role in interpreting the location and intensity of the pain.

Pain Threshold

It is the lowest intensity of the stimulus that is recognised as pain. The threshold of the pain is approximately the same in all normal individuals. But dirrerent individuals react differently to pain in clinical situation.

Thus, the pain has two aspects:

(a) Perception of pain (Sensation),

(b) Emotional reaction with perception.

The reaction with perception varies from individual to individual. In some cases, psycological component of the pain may be much more important than the pain stimulus. Under certain situations, the threshold for excitation of the pain fibres becomes progressively lower and lower as the pain stimulus continues and the pain receptors become more activated. This increase in the sensitivity of the pain fibres is called "Hyperalgesia".

Types of Pain

According to the cause, pain can be:

(a) Pricking Pain or Cutting Pain (due to cut, or pricked with pin)

(b) Burning Pain (due to burn or gastric acid in peptic ulcer)

(c) Aching Pain (arising from the deep tissues, it may be felt as cramps in spasm. Aching is not felt at surface)

The pain is also classified on the location of it's origin :

(i) Superficial or Cutaneous Pain (arising from skin, mucus membrane)

(ii) Deep Non-Visceral Pain (originating from joints, muscles, bone)

(iii) Visceral Pain (arising from the internal visceral organs)

The cutaneous pain and deep non-visceral pain are together termed as "Somatic Pain".

Causes of Pain

The pain can be caused due to Ischemia, Inflammation, Muscle spasm and direct stimulation which can be due to irritation.

Headache and Facial Pain

Headache is the most frequent form of the pain. In most instance, it is a symptom of tension and fatigue, associated with the stress and strain of every day living. However, headache can also be due to several other causes.

The parenchyma of the brain and the skull are insensitive to pain, but the skin, subcutaneous tissues, muscles, blood vessels, meninges and structures of the eye, ear & nose are sensitive to the pain.

Causes of Headache

Headache are usually caused by :

(i) Dilation, distension, traction, or displacement of cranial blood vessels.

(ii) Compression, traction, or disease of spinal cord or cranial muscles.

(iii) Spasm, inflammation, or trauma of cervical or cranial muscles.

(iv) Raised intracranial pressure or meningeal irritation.

Intracranial tumors cause headache only when they result in displacements, deformity, or traction of blood vessels or meninges.

Types of Headache

The Headache can be -

(i) Tension headache and Psychogenic headache

(ii) Migraine

(iii) Cluster headache

(iv) Headache associated with brain tumour and raised intra cra nial pressure.

(v) Headache associated with meningeal irritation

(vi) Vascular headache

(vii) Referred headache

(ix Facial pain associated with neuralgias.

(x) Due to Herpes zoster.

Fever or Pyrexia

The Pyrexia is an elevation of the body temperature above normal, due to disturbances in the temperature regulating mechanism.

The normal body temperature varies from person to person between 97^0 F to 99^0 F, Commonly, by normal body temperature is meant 98.6^0 F (about 37^0 c).

The "hyperpyrexia" is a condition when the body temperature reaches or exceeds 40.5^0 C (105^0 F)

Receptors

The central receptor is located in the anterior part of Hypothalamus and at periphery mainly located in the skin.

The central part of the Hypothalamus, consists of a group nerve cells that are sensitive to the temperature of the arterial blood flow reaching to them.

Types of Fever

Depending upon the cause & severity of the disease, the Pyrexia conditions can be:

(i) Intermittent- The fever comes down to normal state each day.

(ii) Remittent- The fever comes down every day but does not reach normal.

(iii) Sustained- The fever is persistent without significant variation.

(iv) Replapsing- The febrile periods occur between one or several days.

Causes of Fever

The fever can be caused due to - Infections, Tumour & Infracts, Agranulocytosis, Collagen diseases & Gout, disturbances of the Central Nervous System and Heat Stroke.

Adverse Effects of Fever

(i) It acclerates metabolic activity, and results in protein wastage and body weight loss.

(ii) Pain (Headache), Photophobia and Rigours.

(iii) Significant salt and water loss from the body.

(iv) May cause Cardiac or Cerebral vascular disease, specially in elderly patients.

Machanism of Reducing Body Temperature

When the body temperature tends to rise, there is withdrawal of sympathetic vasoconstrictor activity. Consequently, more blood flows towards the skin and heat is lost. If this machanism does not suffice, the heat regulating centre which is situated in the hypothlamus, promotes sweating and evaporation of sweat, thus facilitating loss of heat. The release of the bradykinin from the sweat glands, induces further vasodilation and heat loss from the body.

Treatment of Pain and Fever

The treatment of fever and pain involves:

(i) Treatment with drugs,

(ii) Physio-therapy,

(iii) Surgical procedures.

Analgesic

The drug which relieve pain are called Analgesics. The analgesics act on the pain centre situated in the brain (probably in the thalamus) . The analgesic drugs are non-narcotic or narcotic analgesics. Most of the analgesics belong to the non-steroidal anti-inflammatory drugs (N.S.A.I.D.'s) except narcotic analgesics and some non-narcotic like Paracetamol. The analgesics inhibit prostaglandin synthesis, there by relieving pain & inflammation.

Antipyretic

The drugs which bring down elevated body temperature to normal are called antipyretic drugs. The antipyretic drugs act on the "heat regulating centre" situated in the hypothalamus of the brain and as a result bring about peripheral vasodilation and sweating, causing heat loss from the body.

Classification of Analgesics

Broadly analgesics are classified into:

(a) Narcotic Analgesics.

(b) Non-narcotic Analgesics.

(a) Narcotic Analgesics

They are possessing only powerful analgesic action. The narcotic analgesics group includes-

(i) Natural Opium Alkaloides e.g. Morphine, Codeine.

(ii) Semisynthetic derivative of Natural Alkaloides e.g. Heroin, Oxymorphine.

(iii) Synthetic e.g. Pethidine & it's derivatives like Dextropropoxyphene.

(iv) Agonist- Antagonist Opioids e.g. Pentazocine.

Pethidine, Morphine, when used cause drowsiness, euphoria, dysphoria, respiratory derpression, reduction of the secretion of gastric acid and digestive enzymes , decrease in intestinal motility, constricition of pupil, smooth muscle spasm, and physical & psychological addiction,etc.

(1) Codeine

The codeine is comparatively a week analgesic, acts only in mild to moderate pain. It diminishes the cough reflex & decreases bowel motility, because of these effects the codeine canbe used as an anti-tussive and as an anti-diarrhoeal.

(2) Dextropropoxyphene (Propoxyphene)

It is the derivative of Methodine, having analgesic action, but weeker than Methodine. It binds to opioid receptors and produces analgesia like other opioid. It is rapidly absorbed & diffuses all over the body. Achieves plasma level within 1 to 2 hours and is excreted mainly through urine.

Propoxyphene exerts very low incidence of side effects. Nausea, vomiting may occur, but in high doses may cause drowsiness, headache, vertigo and addiction.

(3) Pentazocine

Pentazocine possess week narcotic antagonist action. When given through parenteral route exerts very potent analgesic action similar to Morphine, but without causing addiction, so it can be used for a longer period.

Pentazocine is very well absorbed and achieves peak plasma level within 15 minutes to 1 hour after parenteral administration and 1 to 3 hours after oral administration. Mainly excreted through urine. It exerts high incidence of side effects including hallucinations, nightmares, disorientation, bizarre feeling, nausea, vomiting, sedation, respiratory depression and increases in pulmonary artery pressure may occur.

(b) Non-narcotic Analgesics

They are effective against pain of mild to moderate intensity. Most of the non-narcotics exert analgesic, antipyretic and anti-inflammatory action and incomparision to narcotic analgesics having very less side effects. The non-narcotic analgesics includes

(i) Salicylates- Sod. Salicylate, Acetylsalicylic acid (Aspirin), etc.

(ii) Para-Aminophenol derivatives- Phenacetin, Paracetamol (Acetaminophen).

(iii) Pyrazolone derivatives- Phenylbutazone, Oxyphenbutazone, Amidopyrine, Analgin (Metamizol).

(iv) Indole derivatives- Indomethacin.

(v) Propionic acid derivatives- Ibuprofen, Fenoprofen, Ketoprofen, Naproxen, Flurbiprofen.

(vi) Anthranilic Acid derivatives- Mefenamic acid, Flufenamic acid

(vii) Oxicam derivatives- Piroxicam, Tenoxicam.

(viii) Phenyl Acetic acid- Diclofenac.

(ix) Sulfonanilide derivatives- Nimesulide.

(1) Aspirin

The Acetylsalicyclic acid or Aspirin is the most effective & most extensively used Salicylates, having analgesic, antipyretic and anti-inflammatory action. Aspirin exerts analgesic & anti-inflammatory action by inhibiting prostaglandin synthesis (mainly peripherally) and antipyretic action by a central action in the hypothalamic area.

Aspirin after oral administration is rapidly absorbed & achieves peak plasma level in about 2 hours. It is mainly excreted through Kidneys as Salicylic acid and other metabolites, only traces of Salicylates are excreted through sweat, bile and faeces.

The untoward side-effets of Aspirin includes G.I. bleeding peptic ulceration, dyspepsia, partial loss of hearing, dizziness, urticaria, depression of platelets aggregation (due to this property used in low dosage in the management of ischemic heart disease) and metabolic effect in children (contraindicated in the children below 12 years specially having viral fever).

(2) Paracetamol

Paracetamol or Acetaminophen is a metabolite of

Phenacetin. It is a potent analgesic and antipyretic. It inhibits the synthesis of prostaglandin in the central nervous system.

Paracetamol is rapidly & completly absorbed after oral administration and achieves peak plasma level in 30 to 60 minutes. It diffuses from the blood relatively uniformly to the most tissues and body fluids. Mainly excerted through urine.

Paracetamol is to be practically free from the toxic side effects, some time nausea, vomiting may occur. The hypersensitivity reactions are quite rare and hepatic toxicity also occurs very rarely, only in very high dose (10 to 20 gm/day). Hence, as an analgesic and antipyretic for day to day use, Paracetamol has become popular.

(3) Ibuprofen

Ibuprofen is basically a Phenylpropionic acid derivatives, possesses potent anti-inflammatory, mild analgesics, and week anti-pyretic action. Their exact mechanism of action is unknown,although its analgesic and anti-inflammatory effect is due to inhibition of prostaglandin synthesis in inflammatory tissues by acting on enzyme, Cyclo -Oxygenase.

Ibuprofen is rapidly absorbed from the G.I.tract and achieves peak plasma level in 90 minutes after an oral dose on an empty stomach. Its half life is about 2 hours and mostly excreted in the urine.

The side effects includes nausea, diarrhoea, G.I. bleeding, rashes, sweating,drowsiness, diziness, peripheral oedema, bruising & blood dyscrasias may occur. It is contra-indicated in peptic-ulcer, asthamatic attack and to the patients having hypersensitivity with the drug.

Ibuprofen in combination with Paracetamol are now widely used for better therapeutic results and tolerance.

(4) Diclofenac

It is a derivative of Phenylacetic acid, shows a high degree of anti-inflammatory, analgesic & antipyretic activity. It inhibits prostaglandin synthesis in inflammatory tissues by acting on Cyclo-Oxygenase & Lypoxygenase enzymes.

Diclofenac is rapidly & efficiently absorbed after oral administration and achieve peak plasma concetration in about 2 hrs. & about 4 hours in the synovial fluid. It is eliminated mainly through urine & to lesser extent through bile as metabolite. Given orally as BID or TID dose. It is highly bound to serum protein, mainly the albumin.

Diclofenac is free from addiction or habbit formation. The undesirable effects are occasional epigastric pain, nausea, vomiting, anorexia, flatulance, dyspepsia, diarrohoea, headache, dizziness, vertigo, rashes, skin eruptions may occur. Rarely G.I. bleeding, drowsiness or urticaria can occur. It is contra-indicated in active peptic ulcer, GI. bleeding and NSAID induced allergic asthma cases.

Diclofenac raises the level of B-endorphin in the blood, so pain is not felt. Diclofenac sodium and Diclofenac potassium are used alone, or in combination with Paracetamol for better therapeutic results.

(5) Piroxicam

Piroxicam is an Oxicam derivative with potent analgesic and anit-inflammatory effects. It is a potent inhibitor of prostaglandin synthesis through reversible inhibition of the Cyclo-Oxygenase enzyme and inhibits migration and aggregation of leucocytes & monocytes in the area of inflammation. It also inhibits release of lysosomal hydrolases as well as the generation of superoxide anions.

Piroxicam is rapidly & nearly completely absorbed and obtains peak plasma level in about 2 hours following oral administration. After absorption, is preferentially disributed in inflamed & damaged tissues and synovial fluid. The elimination half life of Piroxicam is extended due to a low renal clearance rate and is approximately 45 hours. It requires a convenient once daily dose for therapeutic response.

Possible adverse effects are mainly gastric irritation (including nausea, stomatitis, anorexia, constipation, flatulence, ,abdominal pain or diarrhoea), peripheral oedema, ocular irritation and some times hypersensitivity reaction. It is contra-indicated in peptic ulcer syndrome, renal dysfunction, bronchial asthma & to the patients having hypersensitivity to the drug.

(6) Nimesulide

Nimesulide is a Sulfonanilide derivative with potent anti-inflammatory, analgesic and anti-pyretic properties. It inhibits prostaglandin synthesis in inflamed tissues and has relatively little effect on prostaglandin synthesis in organs like the stomach, lungs and kidneys unlike other NSAID's. It also inhibits histamine release from the mast cells. Besides it also reduces superoxide formation within the neutrophils and protects anti-trypsin and thus successfully prevents destructive action of elastase an enzyme produced by neutrophils. Nimesulide, by a direct scavenging action reduces the extracellular concentration of highly toxic hypochlorous acid.

After oral administration of Nimesulide, more than 80% is rapidly absorbed which is not affected by the presence of food. The peak plasma concentration is reached between 2 to 3.2 hours with a half life of 4 hours. Nimesulide is 99% bound to plasma proteins and excreted mainly by the kidneys and to lesser extent through the faeces.

The side effects are usually mild & mainly related to G.I. system and CNS including-gastric pain, nausea, vomiting, hyperchlorhydria, drowsiness, vertigo, insomnia, urticaria & exanthema may occur sometimes. It is contra-indicated in peptic ulcer, moderate to severe hepatic impairment.

(7) Mefenamic Acid

Mefenamic Acid exerts peripheral as well as central analgesic action that does't interfere with uricosuric action of Sulphinpyrazone, therefore, useful in Gout. It also has anti-inflammatory and antipyretic actions. It is commonly used for all painful musculo-skeletal condition and fabrile conditions.

The side effects are usually mild and mainly related to G.I. System (diarrhoea, epigastric distress), skin rashes, dizziness and haemolytic anaemia. It is contra-indicated in epilepsy, glaucoma, G.I. bleeding and to the patients having hypersensitivity with the drug.

Section- B

CHAPTER- 17

Inflammation and Immunity

Pathology

Pathology means study of a disease. It includes the cause of disease and the changes it brings about in the structure and function of cells, tissues, organs and systems. The study of cause of disease is known as "Aetiology".

Types of Diseases

The diseases can be:

(i) Congenital Diseases

The diseases or defects which are present from the birth are termed "Congenital". For example Club foot, Hare lip are Congenital deformities.

(ii) Acquired Diseases

The diseases or defects which develop later in the life are termed as "Acquired". For example Bacterial infections, Scurvy, Cancer, Fracture etc. are Acquired diseases.

(iii) Hereditary or Inherited Disorders

They are those that are passed by parents to their offspring by way of genetic endowment. The hereditary or inherited disorders may be manifested at birth, or remain dormant for sometimes and exhibit themselves later. For example Sickle Cell Anaemia, Haemophilia etc. are Inherited disorders.

Common Causes of Diseases

The most common causes of diseases are as written below:

(i) Injury- They are called traumatic disorders caused due to trauma or injury, e.g.- Burns, Wounds, Fractures.

(ii) Infection- It is the succesful invasion, establishment and growth of the living organisms in the tissue of the host. They may be Viruses, Bacteria, Protozoa, or Helminths.

(iii) Immunological- The interactions between antigens and antibodies, e.g. Allergy, Rheumatoid arthritis.

(iv) Metabolic- The deficiency or excess of a vitamin, an enzyme, a hormone due to derangement of metabolism, e.g.Gout, Diabetes mellitus, Rickets.

(v) Vascular- Vascular changes can lead to disease conditions due to impaired blood supply, e.g.Angina Pectoris.

(vi) Tissue Growth- The excess growth of cells gives rises to tumour (Neoplasm), which may be benign or malignant, e.g. Carcinoma.

Effects of Disease

The effects of the disease may be functional, structural or both. They may be seen at the level of cell, tissues, organs, systems and finally the whole body. For example Necrosis (cellular death) due to serious damage by disease to cells, Hyperplasia (more formation) in the leukaemia, the cancer of blood, Hypoplasia(less formation) of an organ as in the case of some women's ovaries, Oedema (accumulation of water& salt) and Congestive Heart Failure due to hypertension.

Inflammation

Inflammation means reaction of the living tissue to injury, irritation, or infections. The causative factors may be physical such as heat, chemical such as acid or an alkali, or biological such as a bacterium or a virus.

The inflammation can be:

(i) Simple Inflammation- There is no flow of pus or other products of inflammation.

(ii) Acute Inflammation- It may develop rapidly and run a short, stormy course, e.g. Pneumonia.

(iii) Chronic Inflammation- It may develop slowly and run a long course with alternating periods of quiescence and activity, e.g. Tuberculosis.

The term used to described inflammation of a tissue or an organ usually end with the suffix-"ittis" following the organ's name in Greek, Latin or English, for example the inflammation of Conjunctiva termed as "Conjunctivitis", the inflammation of joints termed as "Arthritis" and the inflammation of Oesophagus termed as "Oesophagitis".

Signs and Symptoms of Inflammation

(i) Redness (Robor)

(ii) Swelling (Tumor)

(iii) Pain (Dolor)

(iv) Heat (Calor)

(v) Loss of the function.

Pathology of Inflammation

During the course of inflammation there are two types of changes that occur in the body-Vascular and Cellular.

Vascular Changes

When ever the tissues or cells are damaged, they release Histamine & Histamine like substances which in turn cause relase of Prostaglandins. The Prostaglandins are vasodilator hence changing vasscular permeability, so more blood flows (hyperaemia) through the affected tissue resulting redness (Rober). The dilated capillaries become more permeable & allow the plasma to escape into the intracellular tissue space resulting into swelling (Tumor).

The swelling in turn puts pressure on the local sensory nerve ending thereby causing pain (Dolor). Since increased blood flow brings more heat (Calor) to the inflammed tissue, it feels warmer to touch than the neighbouring tissue. Lastly, inflammation often impairs the function of the affected tissue.

Cellular Changes

It comprises the migration of W.B.C.'s through the wall of dilated capillaries into the affected tissue spaces in an attempt to destroy the micro-organisms. The collection of plasma, white blood cells and /or bacteria which form at the site of inflammation is called "inflammatory exudate".

Inflammation is a protective reaction of the body. However, inflammation can sometimes be harmful either because it is far more severe and extensive than is necessary to dispose of the irritant, or because it is a misdirected response of the body's own tissues (e.g.Rheumatoid arthritis). So in these conditions it needs to be suppressed with the drugs (For drugs see Chapter 2 and 16 of this Section).

Prostaglandins

In 1936 Prostaglandins were isolated from the Seminal fluid. They are synthesized in almost all body cells. During injury to the tissues, there are some chemical changes which takes place in the body and a substance known as Phospholipids is released, Phospholipids converted into Arachiodonic acid in excess quantity, combine with enzymes Cyclo-Oxygenase (mainly) and Lypoxygenase to release Prostaglandins.

Prostaglandins are classified into classes like:

Pg-G, E, F, H, I, A, B, C, and D. The Prostaglandins bind to specific receptor sites present on cells and act locally. Prastaglandins have an important role to play in inflammations and pain cycle of the body.

Oedema

It is the accumulation of fluid in the tissue spaces. It may be localised to a part of the body or it may be generalised (anasarca).

Local oedema is caused by inflammation, allergy, or congestion due to venous thrombosis. The generalised oedema results from a disease of the Liver (Hepatic Oedema), Heart (Cardiac Oedema), Kidney (Renal Oedema), or from gross malnutrition (Nutritional Oedema). The ultimate mechanism of oedema is increased formation and diminished reabsorption of tissue fluid.

Immunity

The immunity means non-susceptibility due to the presence of adequate defensive mechanism in the body against infection.

The immune system is composed of the Lymphatic vessels and Lymphnodes, Thymus gland, Spleen, Liver and White Blood Cells. It has been demonstrated that the body responds to a variety of complex substances in the same way as it does to micro-organisms, by producing "antibodies" and "Sensitised Lymphocytes".

The antibodies are protein in nature (Globulins) and are produced by plasma cells. They develop in the body due to the introduction of foreign (Proteins or Protein Conjugates) substances called "antigens" in the body. Some substances behave as antigens only when coupled with a protein and are called "haptens". Antigen and antibodies show a high degree of specificity, i.e. an antibody will react only with the antigen or hapten which induced it.

The antibodies are also known as " immunoglobulins " (Ig). Most of the immunoglobins are concerned with immunity and are called "protective antibodies" (IgG), where as a certain variety of immunoglobin is also responsible for the adverse antigen-antibody reactions like anaphylactic shock and are called "reaginic antibody" (IgE).

In general, the body responds immunologically only to the foreign substances, not to its own components. However, sometimes the body shows an immunological response to the self tissues, either because of the tissue has undergone some change or because its memory fails . In these conditions, the antibodies and sensitised Lymphocytes that are formed cause damage to the tissue or the organ concerned. This is known as "autoimmunity ", and the disease arsing from it is known as "autoimmune disorders". For example Rheumatoid Arthritis, Rheumatic Fever.

Immune Response

The activity of sensitised Lymphocytes in dealing with antigens is known as "immune response". The sensitised Lymphocytes which are produced by lymph nodes and produce antibodies are called " B-Lymphocytes", where as the sensitised Lymphocytes which are produced by Thymus, are called "T-Lymphocytes". The T-Lymphocytes which help B-Lymphocytes to produce antibodies are called " helper cells", and other don't help B-Lymphocytes to produce antibodies are called "suppressor cells".

The immune response is of two types- "Humoral (Chemical) Immune Respose" and "Cellular Immune Response". The process by which B-lymphocytes produces antibodies by combining with antigen and destroying it is called Humoral Immune Response. The Humoral Immune Response can work against the body and may give rise to allergy.

The process by which T-Lymphocytes destroy the foreign organisms/ substances is called Cellular Immune Response, e.g.

Grafting or transplantion of tissue /organ into the body from another individual can produce adverse effects.

Hypersensitivity or Allergy

It means all sorts of unpleasant or harmful reactions manifested in the body due to sensitivity to substances called "allergens". The allergens are foreign (Protein or Protein Congugates) substances or sometimes drugs or certain other things, which may also produce allergy. So we can say that allergies are a reaction to allergens.

Common allergies at home are caused due to dust mites, animal hairs, insect bites, milk, egg, fish, pollen spores, artificial jewellery, chemicals or tiny creatures.

The allergic reactions occur due to the liberation of "Histamine or Histamine like substance " by the body cells, called " Mast Cells". The Histamine receptor cells are of two types H_1 receptor (Found in the skin, lung tissue, intestinal mucosa), and H_2 receptor (found in the stomach). The H_1 receptor cell stimulation results in the allergic manifestations. Histamine causes vasodilation, mucus glands to secrete and contraction of smooth muscles.

Once a person's body has produced antibody, any future exposure to some allergen will stimulate antibody production in the person's body.

The allergic or hypersensitivity reactions can be Common allergic reaction, Anaphylactic reaction, Cytolytic reaction, Toxic complex reaction or Delayed cell-medicated reaction. The "Anaphylactic Shock" is a condition of emergency where the patient suddenly gets the severe shock on injection of foreign protein (even in a very small dose). If not treated promptly, it can be fatal. The treatment of Anaphylactic Shock involves use of Inj.Adrenaline and /or Inj. Corticosteroid preparations {Inj. Dexona (Cadila H.C.), Inj. Decdan (Merind), Inj. Wymesome (Wyeth), Wycort (Wyeth), etc.}

Common Anti Allergic Drugs

The common anti-allergic drugs are of four main types as written below:

(i) Antihistamines

These are most commonly used for counteracting the allergic reactions or manifestations. The antihistamines act by blocking the action of Histamine (H_1 receptor). The most common side effects of antihistamine are drowsiness (except with Astemizole, Terfenadine, Loratidine) and dryness of the mouth.

(ii) Adrenergic Drugs or Sympathetic Activator Drugs

These are now not commonly used.

(iii) Corticosteroids

These are the most potent anti-allergic agents. Steroids reverse the allergic phenomena by blocking the intracellular production of Histamine or Histamine like substances by sensitized cell. This is made possible as steroid inhibits the antibodies production, as a result preventing antigen-antibody reaction and thus the allergy.

The adverse effects of steroids are indigestion, acne, weight gain, muscle weakness, fluid retention, depression and mood changes.

(iv) Sodium Cromoglycate

It is belived to act by preventing the release of Histamine or Histamine like substances from the mast cells. Used commonly as spray inhaler for the prevention of asthmatic attacks, nasal drops for allergic rhinitis and eye drops for allergic conjunctivitis.

For common anti-allergic drugs, See Chapter 8 and 11 of this section.

Section- B

Chapter- 18

Phytopharmaceuticals

Ayurveda

"Artharveda" is an old Hindu scriptures described the fundamental principals of "Ayurveda". The word Ayurveda is composed of two words:

Ayur = Life

Veda = Knowledge

So Ayurveda is the knowledge or science of life. Here life menas integration of body (Sharira), perceptory organ (Indriyas), mind (Satwa) and soul (Atma). Hence Ayurveda is not only treating ailing body but also considers every aspects of the life.

Ayurveda is based on a principal of "Tridosha" and they are- "Vata", "Pitta" and "Kapha". The vata deals with the functions of nervous system i.e. Central and Autonomic nervous system. The pitta deals with the functions of metabolism and utilisation. And the kapha is responsible for the nourishment and regeneration of all kinds of cells and tissues of the body.

In any living organism, all the three doshas are present. An ideal balance between these elements is responsible for health or "Prakriti" and any disharmony or imbalance among these three doshas contribute to the ill health or "Vikriti".

Depending upon prakriti, these doshas, types differ in health, in emotions or adjustment to disease. So an Ayurvedic formulation must be worked out in such a way that will bring back the dosha combination to an ideal balance.

Just like three doshas of the body, the mind has "Trigunas" and they are "Satwa"(conciousness or knowledge),"Rajas" (motion or action) and "Tamas" (inertia). These three gunas are manifested in the human beings in their temperament, constitution and behaviour which constitute the personality of the being i.e. "Manas Prakriti".

Traditional Ayurvedic medicines are based on various pathas given in ancient scriptures, but in modern lifestyle, for a busy physician these all may be impracticable. Therefore in modern Ayurvedic formulations, efforts are always made to include all the useful constituent ingredients to bring back all the three doshas in an ideal balance.

The Ayurvedic market segment is growing at an encouraging rate,with renewed interest not only amongst modern physicians, but also amongst literate class of society in this ancient method of the treatment, with the formulations suited for the current conditions.

The large interest of the public pave the way for Phyto-Pharmaceuticals, to come into the modren medicine market.

Phyto-Pharmaceuticals

It means preparing (formulating) medicines from the plants.

The man is much indebted to plants. The plants oxygenate the air and favourably influence climatic conditions for him. The plants also continue to provide nourishment for his well being. Moreover, plants also served and will continue to serve as an inexhaustible reservoir of medicines to provide relief from his diverse ailments.

In the early and medieval days man's dependence upon the medicines was entirely on the nature. Through exhaustive observation and studies, with the resources then available, the plants medicine system got organised in different parts of the world including India. The system of medical practice in India, as documented in the "Charak Samitha" and the "Sushruta Samitha" well before the time of Christ, laid emphasis not only on diseases, their symptoms and diagnosis but also on individualised patient approach in treatment.

The basis of herbal medicines was based on their beneficial effects on the symptoms and course of the disease. The modes of action or pharmacological effects of these medicines however, were largely unknown.

The discovery and development of synthetic pharmaceuticals changed the primary dependence of man on nature for his medical requirements. Experimentally and clinically established pharmacological actions of synthetic drugs to eradicate or manage disease provide a logical basis for their World wide acceptance and as a result phyto-therapy (Ayurvedic) has declined sharply especially in the developed countries, where as still Ayurveda is a major therapeutic resource in non urban areas of the developing countries.

Recent years however, have witnessed a renewed interest in plants as a source of valuable and useful medicines. Several reasons evidently, have contributed to this. These include:-

(i) Safety in all age group compared to the synthetic medicines.

(ii) Identification of pharmacological activities in some plants.

(iii) To avoid possible chemical pollution due to the extensive use of synthetic medicines.

(iv) Relative limitation of synthetic medicines, as most of the available drugs (except antimicrobials, vaccines and synthetic vitamins) donot cure the underlying diseases though they may exert prompt favourable effects on signs and symptoms, and so on.

The out come of this changes, is the association of herbal medicines along with specific chemotherapy or completely phytotherapy in certain disease conditions. The new approach to herbal medicines is receiving increasing support from the modren medical profession in many countries (including developed countries).

Phytotherapy also has undergone changes. The metaphysical, sociocultural and traditional aspects of phytotherapy are being replaced by a more systemic pharmacotherapy based on the pharmacological effects of plants or chemical substances isolated from the plants.

To study phytochemicals, much work has been done in this direction during the past few decades and much more well planned studies are underway. These studies are undertaken to determine the main plants chemical group(s), its invitro and in animal effects to establish pharmacological properties and clinical usefulness.

The phytochemical studies have identified a number of medically useful properties and chemical substances in plants which can be of considerable therapeutic potential with obvious advantages. These activities are summarised below:-

(i) Antibacterial, Antiviral and Antifungal activites.

(ii) Hepatoprotective and Choleratic actions (synthetic drugs with hepatoprotective effects are not yet available)

(iii) Anti-inflammatory and antirheumatic activity.

(iv) Cardiovascular activity (Antihypertensive, antiarrythmic & cardiotonic action)

(v) Antiseptic and action on gastroduodenal mucus membrane, to be useful as an adjunct in peptic ulcer management.

(vi) Rich source of natural Vitamins and minerals

(vii) Pharmacological action on benign Prostatic hypertrophy.

Besides, a number of other useful pharmacological actions such as analgesic, antiallergic, antiasthma, hypoglycemic, carminative, appetiser, digestive, laxative, action on uterus, nervine tonics, diuretic and rejuvenator activities have been reported by investigators studying medicinal plants.

Though more clinical studies are required in this direction, but the potential value of Phytopharmaceuticals is amply clear from the investigations already under taken.

Applied Medicines

Now- a- days large number of Phytopharmaceutical products are available in the market for the treatment of various diseases/ disorders.

Few of them are as summerised below:

(1) Anti-infective-

Septilin (Himalaya), Neeri(Aimil), Bangshil (Alarsin)

(2) Cerebral stimulants and activators-

Mentat (Himalaya), Ginkocer (Ranbaxy), Remembre (Biona), Neurotone (Reliance), Mega Mind 2 Plus (Dalmia), Ginvas (C.F.L.)

(3) Enzymes and carminatives-

Gastrozyme (Reliance), Gasex (Himalaya), Ojus (Charak), Satimuliv (Franco), Elcarim (TTK), Bonnisan (Himalaya), Satizym (Twilight), Livotone (East India).

(4) Hepatobillary preparations-

Liv-52 (Himalaya), Tefroli (TTK), Triveng (Rallis), Livoerb (Alkem)

Hepatogard (Themis Ph.), Hepax (Anglo Fr.), Lycovin (Lyka), Tonactive (Lupin), Livomyn (Charak), Vimliv (Dey's), Adliv (Albert David), Nirocil (Solumik), Amlycureds (Aimil), Livex (Ban Labs).

(5) Luxatives, Purgatives and Lubricants-

Nature care (Dabur), Herbolax (Himalaya), Regulax (Charak), Smooth (Biona), Naturolax (Inter Care), Softvac (Lupin), Evacuol (Franco), Igol (Raptakos), Isogel (Allenburys).

(6) Tonics, Rejuvenator, vitamins and Minerals-

One Be (Lupin), Revital (Ranbaxy), Biovital (Micro), Trinergic (Unichem), Virilex (TTK), Mannol (Charak), Ginsec (Duphar), Jensheng (BE), Winofit Ginseng (Wockhardt), Vitalyf (Twilight), Libidol (Natura), Young & Fit (Biona), Gintona (Lyka), Mansex (Reliance), Dassh (ThemisChem.), Amyron (Aimil), Bio-E (Natura), Vitton-99 (Ban Labs).

(7) Hypoglycaemics-

Diat-Aim (Tide), Nosulin (Dey's), Diabecon (Himalaya).

(8) Anti-inflammatory drugs and topical analgesics-

Cerrata plus (Reliance), Tab. Rumalaya (Himalaya), R-compound (Alarsin), Cream-Rumalaya (Himalaya), Metacin Pain Balm(Themis Ph.).

(9) Diuretics and renal calculus-

Aluretic (Alarsin), Cystone (Himalaya), Calcury (Charak), Calursion (Ban Labs).

(10) Drugs for Prostatic hypertrophy-

Prostina (Dey's)

(11) Cough Mixtures-

Dr's Keffs (Biona), Dekofcyn (Alarsin), Jufex (Aimil), Honeytus (Dabur), Crux (Ban Labs).

(12) Antistress drugs-

Geriforte (Himalaya), Siledin (Alarsin).

(13) Antihypertensives-

Arjin (Alarsin), Abana (Himalaya).

(14) Haemostatics-

Ayapon (Alarsin), Possex Forte (Charak).

(15) Drugs acting on the uterus-

Mensulin (Search), R.C.Plus (Reliance), M-2 Tone (Charak), Aleos Compound (Alarsin).

(16) Fertility agents-

Mamsa Forte (Raliance), Speman (Himalaya), Fortage (Alarsin).

(17) Drugs for leucorrhoeas-

Lukol (Himalaya), Lukure (TTK), Lucoril (Reliance), Amycordil (Aimil), Myron (Alarsin), Lucogyl (Ban Labs).

(18) Drugs for lactation and post-natal care-

Lactare (TTK), Leptaden (Alarsin).

(19) Drugs for dental care-

Tab. G32 (Alarsin), Co-Q-Dent gel (Lupin).

(20) Drugs for haemorrhoids and anal fissure-

Pilex (Himalaya), Rilo-Forte (Reliance).

(21) Tranqillizers-

Nervomine (Franco), Anxicalm (Lupin).

Section- B

CHAPTER- 19

Medical Terminology

The medical terms are dificult to understand, spell, pronounce and remember, as they are composed of by many dirrerent types of Latin, Greek and English words. It would be impossible to remember all of them after one reading or even after many reading. However, after repeated readings it is possible to remember at least few of them and therefore such an attempt should be made later.

The key to understanding them is the habit of analysing words, i.e.breaking them into their component roots. For example, the word Pneumonitis is made up of two components, viz. Pneumo = Lung (a Noun) and itis (a suffix) = inflammation, thus Pneumonitis means inflammation of the lungs. Take the word Hyperemesis means excessive vomiting and the word Endocarditis, Endo = inner (a prefix), cardia = heart (a noun), itis = inflammation (a suffix), thus endocarditis means inflammation of the inside of the heart.

So we find that medical terms contain either :

a noun, a prefix & a suffix, or a noun, a suffix

or a prefix, a suffix, or a noun, a prefix.

The lists of nouns, prefixes and suffixes are summarised below:

(1) Nouns

adeno	=	gland
aesthesia	=	sensation
algesia	=	pain
angio	=	blood vessel

arthro	=	joint
bleph	=	eyelid
broncho	=	windpipe (bronchi)
cardio	=	heart
capro	=	wrist
cephalo	=	head
cervico	=	neck (cervix)
cheil	=	lip
chole	=	bile
chondro	=	cartilage
coli	=	bowel
costo	=	rib
cranio	=	skull
cysto	=	bladder, sac
cyto	=	cell
dent	=	tooth
derma	=	skin
dypsia	=	thirst
encephalo	=	brain
entero	=	intestine
feto	=	fetus
gastro	=	stomach
genito	=	genitals
glosso	=	tongue
glyco	=	sugar
gnosis	=	knowledge
haemo	=	blood
hepato	=	liver
histo	=	tissue
hydro	=	water
hystero	=	uterus
ictero	=	jaundice
kerato	=	cornea

kinesis	=	movement
lingua	=	tongue
lipo	=	fat
logos	=	study
meningo	=	meninges
metro	=	uterus
myo	=	muscle
nephro	=	kidney
neuro	=	nerve
odonto	=	tooth
oma	=	tumour
onycho	=	nail
opthalmos	=	eye
oro	=	mouth
osteo	=	bone
oto	=	ear
paresis	=	weakness
patho	=	disease
penia	=	deficiency
phagia	=	appetite, eating
pharmaco	=	drug
phlebo	=	vein
pneumo	=	lung
pnoea	=	breathing
procto	=	anus
psycho	=	mind
pyo	=	pus
rhino	=	nose
salpingo	=	fallopian tube
somato	=	body
steato	=	fat
sthenia	=	strength
stoma	=	mouth

trophy = nourishmen

(2) Prefixes

a	=	without, not
ab	=	away from
abdomino	=	abdominal
acro	=	exremity
ad	=	near to (towards)
amphi	=	on both sides,around
an	=	not, without
anti	=	against
auto	=	self
bi	=	twice, two
brady	=	slow
cata	=	down
circum	=	around
co	=	together
contra	=	against
de	=	away from, reversing
di	=	two
dis	=	separation
dys	=	painful, abnormal
ecto	=	out side
em	=	in
endo	=	within, inner
epi	=	on, above, upon
ery	=	red
eu	=	well, normal
exo	=	away from, out of
fore	=	before, in front of
hemi	=	half
hetro	=	unlikness, dissimilarity
hexa	=	six
homeo	=	like

hyper	=	above, excessive
hypo	=	below, less
idio	=	peculiar to the individual
in	=	not, into
infra	=	below, lower
inter	=	between
intra	=	within
intro	=	inward
iso	=	equal
lepto	=	thin, soft
leuko	=	white
macro	=	large
mal	=	abnormal, poor
medi	=	middle
mega	=	large
meno	=	about menses
meta	=	between
micro	=	small
mio	=	smaller
mono	=	one, single
muco	=	mucus
multi	=	many
neo	=	new
oligo	=	less, deficiency
ortho	=	straight
pan	=	all
para	=	beside
peri	=	around
poly	=	many
post	=	after
pre/pro	=	before
pseudo	=	false
quadri	=	four

re = again, back
retro = behind
sclero = hard
semi = half
sub = below
super/supra= above
syn = together, union
tachy = fast
tetro = four
tri = three
uni = one
xanth = yellow
xero = dry

(3) Suffixes

able = capable of
aemia = presence in blood
agra = attack, severe pain
algia = pain
ase = catalyst, enzyme
asis = condition
blast = cell
cele = tumour, swelling
cide = kiling
coccus = spherical cell
cule = little
cyte = cell
dynia = pain
ectasis = dilation
ectomy = removal of
emesis = vomiting
genic = causing
iasis = state, condition of
itis = inflammation

kinesis	=	motion
lysis/lytic	=	breaking down, dissolution
malacia	=	softening
megaly	=	enlargement
oma	=	tumour
osis	=	condition, excess
ostomy	=	toform an opening
pathy	=	disease
penia	=	lack of
phagia	=	swallowing
phasia	=	speech
philia	=	affinity for, liking
phobia	=	fear
plasty	=	repair
pnoea	=	breathing
poiesis	=	making
ptosis	=	falling
rhagia	=	to brust forth
rhoea	=	excessive discharge
stasis	=	cessation of movement
tomy	=	cutting

Abbreviations

BAMS	=	Bachelor in Ayurvedic Medical Science
BDS	=	Bachelor of Dental Surgery
BIMS	=	Bachelor of Indian Medical Science
BP	=	British Pharmacopoeia
DA	=	Diploma in Anaesthesia
DCH	=	Diploma in Child Health
DGO	=	Diploma in Gynaecology and Obstertics
DLO	=	Diploma in Laryngology and Otology
DM	=	Docterate in Medicine
DOMS	=	Diploma in Opthalmic Medicine and Surgery
D.Ortho	=	Diploma in Orthopaedics
DRCOG	=	Diploma in the Royal College of Obst. and Gyn.
DTCD	=	Diploma in Tuberculosis and Chest Disease
DVD	=	Diploma in Venereal Diseases
FACC	=	Fellow of the American College of Cardiology
FACP	=	Fellow of the American College of Physicians
FRCP	=	Fellow of the Royal College of Physicians
FRCS	=	Fellow of the Royal College of Surgeons
GAMS	=	Graduate in Ayurvedic Medical Science
GP	=	General Practitioner
IMA	=	Indian Medical Association
IP	=	Indian Pharmacopoeia
MAMS	=	Member of the Association of Medical Science
MBBS	=	Bachelor of Medicine and Bachelor of Surgery

MD	=	Doctor of Medicine
MDS	=	Master of Dental Surgery
MRCP	=	Member of the Royal College of Physicians
MRSH	=	Member of the Royal Society of Health
MS	=	Master of Surgery
PMO	=	Principal Medical Officer
RMP	=	Registered Medical Practitioner
SMO	=	Senior Medical Officer
USP	=	United State Pharmacopoeia
WHO	=	World Health Organization

Medical Specialities

Broadly the specialities of medical practice can be divided into Medical, Surgical, and Para-Clinical.

(a) Medical Specialities

The most important is 'General Medicines' or "Internal Medicines' and has developed further to superspecialities, viz.- Cardiology, Neurology, Gastroenterology, Nephrology, Endocrinology, Chest-Medicines, Rheumatology, Anaesthesiology.

The other medical specialities are - Paediatrics, Dermatology, Psychiatry, Venereology, Oncology, etc.

(b) Surgical Specialities

The most important is "General Surgery" and has developed further to superspecialities, viz.-Neurosurgery, Plastic Surgery, Urology, Cardiovascular Surgery.

The other surgical specialities are- Gynaecology & Obstertics, Ophthalmology, Orthopaedics, Otorhinolargyngology (ENT).

(c) Para-clinical Specialities

These specialities provides diagnostic facilities. They include Radiology, Pathology, Microbiology, Histopathology & Physiotherapist (include ultra-sonic therapy, etc.).

